Contents

Acetaminophen (Tylenol) 18

Acyclovir (Zovirax) 19

Albuterol (Proventil HFA, ProAir HFA, Ventolin HFA) 20

Alendronate (Fosamax) 21

Allopurinol (Zyloprim) 22

Alprazolam (Xanax) 23

Alteplase (Activase, tPA) 24

Amiodarone (Cordarone) 25

Amitriptyline (Elavil) 26

Amlodipine (Norvasc) 27

Amoxicillin (Amoxil) 28

Amphetamine/Dextroamphetamine (Adderall) 29

Ampicillin/Sulbactam (Unasyn) 30

Aripiprazole (Abilify) 31

Aspirin (Ecotrin) 33

Atenolol (Tenormin) 34

Atomoxetine (Strattera) 35

Atorvastatin (Lipitor) 36

Atropine 38

Azithromycin (Zithromax, Z-Pak) 39

Baclofen (Lioresal) 40

Benazepril (Lotensin) 41

Benzonatate (Tessalon) 42

Benztropine (Cogentin) 43

Bisacodyl (Dulcolax)..44

Bisoprolol (Zebeta)...45

Budesonide – oral (Entocort)....................................46

Bupropion (Wellbutrin, Zyban)................................48

Buspirone (Buspar)...49

Calcium acetate (PhosLo)...50

Carbamazepine (Tegretol)..51

Carbidopa/levodopa (Sinemet)...............................52

Carisoprodol (Soma)...53

Carvedilol (Coreg)..54

Cefazolin (Ancef)..55

Cefdinir (Omnicef)..56

Ceftriaxone (Rocephin)...57

Cefuroxime (Ceftin, Zinacef)....................................58

Celecoxib (Celebrex)...59

Cephalexin (Keflex)...60

Cetirizine (Zyrtec)...61

Ciprofloxacin (Cipro)...62

Citalopram (Celexa)..63

Clindamycin (Cleocin)...65

Clobetasol (Temovate)..66

Clonazepam (Klonopin)...67

Clonidine (Catapres)...68

Clopidogrel (Plavix)..69

Codeine / APAP (Tylenol #3).....................................70

Colchicine (Colcrys)..71

Conjugated Estrogen (Premarin)...............................72

Cyclobenzaprine (Flexeril)..73

Dabigatran (Pradaxa)..74

Darbepoetin alfa (Aranesp).......................................75

Dexlansoprazole (Dexilant).......................................76

Dexmethylphenidate (Focalin)..................................77

Diazepam (Valium)...78

Dicyclomine (Bentyl)..79

Digoxin (Digitek, Lanoxin)..80

Diltiazem (Cardizem CD, Cartia XT)..........................81

Diphenoxylate/atropine (Lomotil).............................82

Divalproex (Valproic Acid, Depakote)........................83

Donepezil (Aricept)..84

Dopamine 85

Doxazosin (Cardura) 86

Doxycycline (Vibramycin) 87

Duloxetine (Cymbalta)..88

Dutasteride (Avodart)...89

Enalapril (Vasotec)...90

Enoxaparin (Lovenox) 92

Epinephrine (EpiPen, Adrenalin) 93

Erythromycin (Ery-tab) 94

Erythropoietin (Procrit, Epogen) 95

Escitalopram (Lexapro)...96

Esomeprazole (Nexium)..98

Eszopiclone (Lunesta) 99

Etanercept (Enbrel)..100

Ethinyl Estradiol and Norgestimate 101

Ezetimibe (Zetia)..102

Famotidine (Pepcid)..103

Febuxostat (Uloric) 104

Fentanyl (Duragesic)..105

Ferrous Sulfate..106

Fexofenadine (Allegra)..107

Filgrastim (Neupogen) 108

Finasteride (Proscar)..109

Fluconazole (Diflucan) 110

Fluoxetine (Prozac) 111

Fluticasone (Flonase) 113

Folic Acid..114

Furosemide (Lasix)..115

Gabapentin (Neurontin) 117

Gemfibrozil (Lopid) 118

Gentamycin..119

Glipizide (Amaryl) 120

Glucagon..121

Glyburide (Micronase, Diabeta) 122

Guaifenesin (Mucinex)..123

Haloperidol (Haldol) 124

Heparin 126

Hydralazine (Apresoline) 127

Hydrochlorothiazide (Hydrodiuril)............................. 128

Hydrocodone/acetaminophen (Norco, Lortab)................... 129

Hydromorphone (Dilaudid) 130

Ibuprofen (Motrin, Advil)...................................... 131

Infliximab (Remicade)... 133

Insulin Aspart (Novolog) 134

Insulin Detemir (Levemir)..................................... 135

Insulin Glargine (Lantus)...................................... 136

Insulin Lispro (Humalog) 137

Irbesartan (Avapro)... 138

Iron sucrose (Venofer).. 139

Ketorolac (Toradol)... 140

Lamotrigine (Lamictal) 141

Lansoprazole (Prevacid)....................................... 142

Latanoprost (Xalatan) 143

Levofloxacin (Levaquin) 144

Levothyroxine (Synthroid) 145

Lisdexamfetamine (Vyvanse)................................... 147

Lisinopril (Zestril, Prinivil) 148

Lithium (Lithobid) 150

Loperamide (Imodium).. 151

Lorazepam (Ativan)... 152

Losartan (Cozaar).. 153

Lovastatin (Mevacor) 154

Meclizine (Antivert) 156

Meloxicam (Mobic) 157

Memantine (Namenda) 159

Metformin (Glucophage) 160

Methadone (Methadose, Dolophine) 161

Methotrexate (Rheumatrex) 162

Methylphenidate (Ritalin, Concerta) 163

Methylprednisolone (Medrol) 164

Metoclopramide (Reglan) 166

Metoprolol succinate (Toprol XL) 167

Metronidazole (Flagyl) 168

Midazolam (Versed) 169

Milk of Magnesia 170

Mirtazapine (Remeron) 171

Mometasone (Nasonex) 172

Montelukast (Singulair) 173

Morphine (MS Contin, Oramorph) 174

Moxifloxacin (Avelox) 175

Nabumetone (Relafen) 176

Naproxen (Naprosyn, Aleve) 178

Nebivolol (Bystolic) 180

Niacin (Niaspan) 181

Nifedipine (Procardia) 182

Nitrofurantoin (Macrobid) 183

Nitroglycerine (Nitrostat) 184

Nitroprusside (Nitropress) 185

Norepinephrine (Levophed) 186

Nortriptyline (Pamelor) 187

Olanzapine (Zyprexa) 188

Olmesartan (Benicar) 190

Olopatadine (Patanol) 191

Omeprazole (Prilosec) 192

Ondansetron (Zofran) 194

Oseltamivir (Tamiflu) 195

Oxybutynin (Ditropan) 196

Oxycodone (Oxycontin, Oxyfast, Oxy IR) 197

Oxycodone/APAP (Percocet) 199

Pantoprazole (Protonix) 201

Paroxetine (Paxil) 202

Pegfilgrastim (Neulasta) 204

Penicillin 205

Phenazopyridine (Pyridium) 206

Phenytoin (Dilantin) 207

Pioglitazone (Actos) 208

Piperacillin/tazobactam (Zosyn) 209

Potassium (Klor-Con) 210

Pramipexole (Mirapex) 211

Pravastatin (Pravachol) 212

Prednisone (Deltasone) 214

Pregabalin (Lyrica) 216

Promethazine (Phenergan) 217

Propofol (Diprivan) 218

Propranolol (Inderal LA) 219

Pseudoephedrine (Sudafed) 220

Quetiapine (Seroquel) 221

Quinapril (Accupril) 223

Rabeprazole (Aciphex) 225

Ramipril (Altace) 226

Ranitidine (Zantac) 228

Rifampin (Rifadin) 229

Risedronate (Actonel) 230

Risperidone (Risperdal) 231

Rivaroxaban (Xarelto) 233

Ropinirole (Requip) 234

Rosuvastatin (Crestor) 235

Sennosides (Senokot) 236

Sertraline (Zoloft) 237

Sildenafil (Viagra) 239

Simvastatin (Zocor) 240

Sitagliptin (Januvia) 242

Spironolactone (Aldactone) 243

Sumatriptan (Imitrex) 244

Tamsulosin (Flomax) 245

Temazepam (Restoril) 246

Terazosin (Hytrin) 247

Testosterone (Androgel, Androderm) 248

Tiotropium (Spiriva) 249

Tolterodine (Detrol LA) 251

Topiramate (Topamax) 252

Tramadol (Ultram) 253

Travoprost (Travatan) 255

Trazodone (Desyrel) 256

Triamcinolone (Kenalog) 257

Triamterene/HCTZ (Dyazide) 258

Trimethoprim/sulfamethoxazole (Bactrim) 259

Valacyclovir (Valtrex) 260

Valsartan (Diovan) 261

Vancomycin (Vancocin) 262

Varenicline (Chantix) 263

Vasopressin (Vasostrict) 264

Venlafaxine (Effexor) 265

Verapamil (Calan) 266

Vitamin D 267

Warfarin (Coumadin, Jantoven) 268

Zolpidem (Ambien) 270

60 Classes in 60 Minutes

5-Alpha Reductase Inhibitors 271

5-HT3 Receptor Antagonists...271

ACE Inhibitors 271

Acetylcholinesterase Inhibitors 271

Alpha Blockers 272

Aminoglycosides...272

Anticoagulants..272

Antiplatelet...272

Antipsychotics...272

ARB's...273

Azole Antifungals 273

Benzodiazepines 273

Beta Blockers 273

Beta-2 Agonists...274

Biguanide 274

Bisphosphonates 274

Calcium Channel Blockers...274

Cardiac Glycosides 275

Cephalosporins 275

COX-2 Inhibitors..275

Dipeptidyl Peptidase-4 Inhibitors 275

DMARDs...276

Dopamine Agonists...276

Erythropoiesis Stimulating Agents.......................................276

Gaba Drugs 276

H1 Blockers, First Generation 277

Histamine Receptor 2 Blockers................................277

HMG-CoA Inhibitors (Statins) 277

Inhaled Anticholinergics 277

Long acting insulins..278

Loop Diuretics..278

Macrolides 278

Miscellaneous Analgesic.......................................279

New Oral Anticoagulants (NOACs) 279

Newer Seizure Meds...279

Nitrates 279

NMDA Antagonist 279

Non-Steroidal Anti Inflammatory Drugs.......................280

Older Seizure Meds 280

Opioids...280

Penicillin's..280

Potassium Sparing Diuretics 281

Prostaglandins 281

Proton Pump Inhibitors 281

Quinolones..281

Rapid Acting Insulins...282

Second Generation Histamine-1 Antagonists....................282

Selective Serotonin & Norepinephrine Reuptake Inhibitors 282

Selective Serotonin Reuptake Inhibitors 283

Skeletal Muscle Relaxants 283

Stimulant Laxatives 283

Stimulants 283

Sulfonylureas 283

Systemic Corticosteroids 284

Thiazide Diuretics 284

Thyroid supplementation 284

Triptans 285

Urinary Anticholinergics 285

Vitamin K antagonist 285

Xanthine Oxidase Inhibitors 285

Z-Drugs 286

Navigating the NCLEX©
Your Insiders' Guide to Nursing Pharmacology

Created by:
Eric Christianson, Pharm.D., BCPS, CGP

Edited by:
Jenna Pakala, Pharm.D.

Copyright and Disclaimer

ABOUT THE AUTHOR

Eric Christianson, Pharm.D., BCPS, CGP is a clinical pharmacist who is passionate about patient safety. Eric is the founder of meded101.com, a website dedicated to providing quality, real world medication education for healthcare professionals. He has been acknowledged by The Wall Street Journal, American Journal of Nursing, National Association Directors of Nursing, Pharmacy Podcast, Pharmacy Today, and Pharmacy Times.

INTRODUCTION

Pharmacology is tough. To improve your chances of passing the NCLEX©, you need to have a basic understanding of pharmacology. I have a deep appreciation of medication mistakes, and understanding pharmacology can save the lives of your patients. I've spent the last 10+ years of my life learning and more importantly applying pharmacology. I've given dozens of presentations on various medication related topics to hundreds of nurses. I've been quoted in the American Journal of Nursing, Wall Street Journal, and my educational website meded101.com is acknowledged on The National Association Directors of Nursing Administration website. I work with nurses daily and understand the struggle of learning pharmacology. I've taken nursing pharmacology in college, and went on to obtain my Pharm.D. from one of the top rated pharmacy schools in the nation. I have a passion for simplifying complex topics and a soft spot in my heart for nurses who do many things that I can't. So, what's special about this study guide?

1. I've taken the top 200+ most commonly prescribed medications and given you ESSENTIAL and RELEVANT information about each of the drugs.
2. To ensure you're prepared for the NCLEX©, I've had nurses who've passed the NCLEX© review the content to provide feedback on what should and shouldn't be included.

3. As a bonus, you get access to the 60 in 60 Study Guide. I breakdown 60 common medication classes with my top 3-5 bullet points that you can get through in 60 minutes or less.
4. The information is relevant to clinical practice. I work with physicians, nurses, and other pharmacists on a daily basis and have learned a ton from them.
5. The medications are all hyperlinked/noted by generic name in the index! This allows for easy access to whichever drug you need to focus. I would recommend learning by generic name as this was recently stated about the NCLEX©, "the NCLEX examination will reflect, on most occasions, the use of generic medication names only"

How should you use this study guide? Drugs can do wacky things to patients. I know it, and I've seen it. However, those "wacky" things that happen once in a career is not what I'm trying to teach you. I'm trying to teach you the stuff that happens daily or should be monitored day after day. Remember, I'm going to provide you the ESSENTIALS to preparing for the NCLEX© and/or your pharmacology courses. This is not intended to be a package insert that lists 45 (exaggeration, but not really) side effects with each medication.

Acetaminophen (Tylenol)

- Class: Analgesic, Antipyretic
- Mechanism of Action: Inhibits prostaglandins in the CNS and may also block pain impulses
- Common Uses: Pain, fever
- Memorable Side Effects: Pretty well tolerated; rash (rare), liver toxicity (rare)
- Clinical Pearls:
  - One of the safest oral medications in the elderly for pain
  - Typically used in pregnancy first line for pain/headaches, etc. if a medication is necessary
  - 4 gram max (possibly 3 gram in elderly/over the counter use)
  - Often found in combo with over the counter and prescription medications; cough and cold products, Vicodin, Percocet etc. (be sure patients are well educated on this to avoid accidental overdose)
  - Liver toxicity extremely rare at recommended doses, usually problem occurs when accidental or intentional overdose happens
  - Acetylcysteine is antidote for acetaminophen overdose

Acyclovir (Zovirax)

- Class: Antiviral
- Mechanism of Action: Inhibits DNA synthesis and viral replication
- Common Uses: Shingles, genital herpes, chicken pox
- Memorable Side Effects: GI most common, CNS side effects more likely in elderly and/or poor kidney function
- Clinical Pearls:
  - Typically for most viral infections, the sooner treatment is started once an infection is identified, the better
  - You can think of acyclovir and valacyclovir as essentially the same...the big advantage of valacyclovir is that patients don't need to take it so many times per day (acyclovir may need to be dosed up to 5 times per day which is far from ideal for our patients)
  - Monitor for GI side effects, and Liver Function Tests will be more important if long term use is necessary
  - May need to reduce dose and/or have a heightened awareness for potential adverse effects in patients with poor kidney function
  - Also comes in a topical form that can be used for cold sores (herpes labialis) or Genital Herpes Simplex Virus

Albuterol (Proventil HFA, ProAir HFA, Ventolin HFA)

- Class: Beta-agonist
- Mechanism of Action: Stimulates beta-2 receptors leading to relaxation of smooth muscle and opening of airways
- Common Uses: Acute relief of respiratory distress in Asthma, COPD
- Memorable Side Effects: tachycardia, tremor, anxiousness
- Clinical Pearls:
  - This medication is the mainstay for an acute asthma exacerbation...i.e. it has a rapid onset and can begin to open up the airway in a few short minutes
  - It is often used with ipratropium (Duoneb/Combivent = brand name)
  - Remember that albuterol (a beta agonist) will have opposite effects of Beta-blockers! Instead of reduced pulse, you could see tachycardia
  - Too much beta-agonist can also be a potential cause of tremor/shakiness
  - In patients who are taking multiple inhaled respiratory medications at the same time, albuterol will be done first to help open up the airways
  - With patients who are frequently using their albuterol inhaler (or nebs) or presenting to the emergency room, make sure that they are reassessed to have their controller (usually inhaled corticosteroids) medication adjusted

Alendronate (Fosamax)

- Class: Bisphosphonate
- Mechanism of Action: Inhibits osteoclasts (osteoclasts break down bone)
- Common Uses: Osteoporosis
- Memorable Side Effects: Esophageal ulceration (administration procedure important to decrease this risk), GI side effects in general
- Clinical Pearls:
  - Timing of administration is critical! Take on an empty stomach, usually right away in the morning with 6-8 ounces of plain water 30 minutes prior to any food or drink (that isn't plain water)
  - Have patient remain sitting or standing upright for 30 minutes (this is to reduce the risk of esophageal irritation or ulceration)
  - Absorption will be limited and drug will not be effective if taken with food or other medications
  - After 3-5 years of bisphosphonate use, some lower risk patients may be able to have the medication reassessed for ongoing need
  - Osteonecrosis (destruction or dying) of the jaw is extremely rare; patients may be at increased risk if recently had an invasive dental procedure
  - Be cautious with oral bisphosphonates in patients who already have esophageal or GI related concerns (GI bleed or ulcer history)
  - Always important to assess adequate vitamin D and calcium intake

Allopurinol (Zyloprim)

- Class: Anti-gout, xanthine oxidase inhibitor
- Mechanism of Action: Inhibits xanthine oxidase and decreases uric acid production
- Common Uses: Decrease uric acid in gout
- Memorable Side Effects: GI issues, rash
- Clinical Pearls:
  - Used for prophylaxis of gout, NOT treatment of an acute flare; NSAIDs, prednisone, or colchicine are generally used for an acute flare
  - Usually fairly well tolerated, but watch out for dose adjustments in CKD; cleared by the kidneys
  - Keep an eye out for medications that can elevate uric acid; niacin, thiazide diuretics

Alprazolam (Xanax)

- Class: Antianxiety, Benzodiazepine
- Mechanism of Action: enhances activity of GABA (an inhibitor neurotransmitter that causes sedation)
- Common Uses: Anxiety, Insomnia
- Memorable Side Effects: sedation, confusion, fall risk, dizziness
- Clinical Pearls:
  - The best way I remember benzodiazepines is that they are very close to "alcohol in a pill"
  - Sedation, slurred speech, confusion, trouble walking (ataxia) etc. are all common with benzo's/alcohol; they are also commonly used in alcohol withdrawal protocols
  - Be cautious with patients on higher doses of benzodiazepines to make sure they aren't abruptly stopped
  - Educate patients on driving/operating machinery (remember that benzodiazepines are often used for sleep as well as anxiety)
  - Flumazenil is antidote in overdose
  - Unlike SSRI's for anxiety, a great advantage of benzo's are that they work quickly and can be used as needed
  - Falls in the elderly is a big downside to using these medications
  - Benzo's are a controlled substance, i.e. they can cause addiction, etc.

Alteplase (Activase, tPA)

- Class: Thrombolytic (clot buster)
- Mechanism of Action: Binds to fibrin and breaks up blood clots
- Common Uses: Stroke, Pulmonary embolism, MI, also can be used to open up central venous access (Cathflo)
- Memorable Side Effects: Bleeding
- Clinical Pearls:
  - Often referred to as tPA
  - Need to use this medication quickly at onset of stroke to have maximal benefit
  - Classified as a thrombolytic (clot buster)
  - Bleed risk is important to monitor – low chance of causing intracranial bleeding, but not good if this happens
  - Extra caution if patients are already receiving anticoagulants (warfarin, dabigatran, etc.)
  - Need to monitor for high blood pressure as this can increase risk of complications

Amiodarone (Cordarone)

- Class: Antiarrhythmic
- Mechanism of Action: Multiple mechanisms including affecting sodium/potassium and calcium channels, as well as potentially having beta and alpha blocking activity
- Common Uses: Atrial fibrillation
- Common Side Effects: Amiodarone can treat arrhythmias, so it can also cause arrhythmias; low blood pressure, GI side effects (nausea, vomiting, anorexia, constipation), hypothyroid, elevated LFT's, pulmonary toxicity
- Clinical Pearls:
    - The usual goal in atrial fibrillation is to control the rate of the heart with beta-blockers or calcium channel blockers (remember only the calcium channel blockers that act on the heart and need to be monitored for pulse – diltiazem and verapamil); Amiodarone is used to control the heart rhythm, not rate, and is usually used second
    - Unique in that it has a very long half-life – it takes about 40-55 days for half of the drug to be eliminated
    - Thyroid function needs to be monitored
    - Respiratory function should be monitored as amiodarone can cause pulmonary fibrosis (it has a black box warning)
    - Liver function needs to be monitored as it has a boxed warning for liver toxicity as well
    - Classic drug interaction with digoxin – end result is that digoxin concentrations can be significantly elevated when amiodarone is started or increased

Amitriptyline (Elavil)

- Class: TCA (tri-cyclic antidepressant)
- Mechanism of Action: Tri-cyclic antidepressant (highly anticholinergic) – inhibits reuptake of serotonin and possibly norepinephrine
- Common Uses: Depression, neuropathy, pain syndromes, anxiety, PTSD
- Memorable Side Effects: Anticholinergic + confusion, fall risk in elderly
- Clinical Pearls:
  - Old TCA generally not recommended in the elderly due to anticholinergic effects
  - Anticholinergic effect = anti – SLUDs; can't salivate, lacrimate, urinate, or defecate OR can't spit, see, pee, or poop
  - In addition, cognitive impairment is not a good thing in the elderly due to possibility of preexisting dementia
  - TCA's may have some benefit in neuropathy, generally much cheaper than SNRI's (duloxetine) which can be also beneficial in neuropathy
  - Not a good first line choice for sleep or depression (other agents exist that are much safer)
  - Look out for TCA's causing the prescribing cascade! Artificial tears for dry eyes, constipation medications, BPH medications like tamsulosin, dementia medications, or artificial saliva

Amlodipine (Norvasc)

- Class: Antihypertensive, Calcium Channel Blocker
- Mechanism of Action: blocks calcium ions from entering voltage smooth muscle, resulting in relaxation (vasodilation) – dihydropyridine calcium channel blocker
- Common Uses: hypertension
- Memorable Side Effects: low blood pressure, edema, constipation
- Clinical Pearls:
  - Very important distinction: You will not see amlodipine used in atrial fibrillation, because its activity is primarily on the vessels; this differs from non-dihydropyridine calcium channel blockers like verapamil and diltiazem that act on the heart AND blood vessels; This also means that pulse monitoring will not be necessary with amlodipine
  - The higher you push the dose on these medications, the more likely you will see the side effect of edema
  - Keep an eye out for new requirement of diuretic Rx's to treat the edema caused by the calcium channel blockers
  - Educate our patients to get up slowly to minimize risk of orthostatic hypotension
  - Amlodipine is usually only dosed once daily which is nice, but you may see it twice daily if the provider feels blood pressure increases as the effects are wearing off
  - Simvastatin is a very common medication that interacts with "most" of the calcium channel blockers, including amlodipine

Amoxicillin (Amoxil)

- Class: Antibiotic, Penicillin
- Mechanism of Action: Inhibits bacterial cell wall formation
- Common Uses: Ear infection, sinusitis, strep throat, skin infections
- Memorable Side Effects: GI side effects most common, allergy, rash
- Clinical Pearls:
  - Many patients have an allergy to penicillin; amoxicillin is from the same class and should not be used in patients with a severe allergy (if it is an intolerance like stomach upset, it may be prudent to try a "penicillin" type antibiotic again depending upon the patient's situation)
  - Diarrhea and GI upset are going to be the major/common side effects with amoxicillin; with mild GI upset and/or diarrhea, hopefully the patient can tough it out and continue therapy
  - Giving amoxicillin with food or a snack may help reduce GI upset
  - We are going to want to monitor the response of the patient, hopefully they will begin feeling better by day 2 or 3 of treatment
  - Temperature would be an important thing to monitor for patients who were significantly febrile
  - If suspension used (common in pediatrics), you must adequately shake to disperse the medication!

Amphetamine/Dextroamphetamine (Adderall)

- Class: CNS Stimulant
- Mechanism of Action: Stimulates release of norepinephrine and dopamine leading to CNS stimulation
- Common Uses: ADHD
- Memorable Side Effects: Anxiety, insomnia, poor appetite, weight loss, hypertension, pulse, emotional lability
- Clinical Pearls:
    - Remembering that this medication ramps you up (stimulant) will help you remember its side effects (anxiety, insomnia, weight loss, poor appetite, increased BP, increased pulse etc.)
    - When used in pediatrics, poor appetite can be a significant problem and should be something that should be assessed
    - BP and Pulse monitoring is important
    - Be cautious in adult patients who may already be at cardiovascular risk (hypertension, etc.)
    - Schedule 2 controlled substance, addictive

Ampicillin/Sulbactam (Unasyn)

- Class: Antibiotic, Penicillin
- Mechanism of Action: Inhibits bacterial cell wall formation
- Common Uses: Endocarditis, Group B strep prevention, sepsis, upper respiratory infections
- Memorable Side Effects: GI side effects most common, allergy, rash
- Clinical Pearls:
  - Be sure to check allergies (don't use if allergic to penicillin, amoxicillin, etc.)
  - Diarrhea and GI upset are going to be the major/common side effects with ampicillin/sulbactam with mild GI upset and/or diarrhea, hopefully the patient can tough it out and continue therapy
  - We are going to want to monitor the response of the patient, hopefully they will begin feeling better by day 2 or 3 of treatment
  - Temperature would be an important thing to monitor for patients who were significantly febrile

Aripiprazole (Abilify)

- Class: Antipsychotic (2nd generation)
- Mechanism of Action: Blocks dopamine receptors
- Common Uses: Schizophrenia, bipolar disorder, depression, dementia related behaviors like aggression, hallucinations, delusions (off-label)
- Memorable Side Effects: Sedation, fall risk, orthostatic BP changes, EPS, metabolic syndrome
- Clinical Pearls:
  - Aripiprazole can be used in patients who have failed traditional monotherapy like SSRI's for depression (usually this is at low doses of aripiprazole)
  - Usually higher doses are required for younger patients with schizophrenia and/or bipolar disorder while lower doses can and should be used in the elderly
  - Remember with antipsychotic medications that they block dopamine and can exacerbate conditions where there is a shortage of dopamine like Parkinson's disorder (remember that we use dopamine to treat Parkinson's – i.e. carbidopa/levodopa)
  - Sedation, orthostatic hypotension, movement disorder side effects can all increase the risk of falls especially in our elderly patients
  - NMS (neuroleptic malignant syndrome) is a very rare but very serious complication with antipsychotic medications; a few symptoms of NMS include: fever, hyperreflexia, confusion, delirium, tremor
  - Antipsychotics increase risk of metabolic syndrome (diabetes, elevated lipids, weight gain etc.) – it is important to periodically monitor for this, especially in younger patients with schizophrenia and/or

bipolar who may be likely to require long term use of higher doses

- ○ Anticholinergic effects are possible as well with antipsychotics, dry eyes, dry mouth, exacerbation of urinary retention (i.e. BPH), constipation (SLUD – can't salivate, lacrimate, urinate or defecate)
- ○ Antipsychotics can contribute to QTc prolongation, which can be especially problematic in patients who are already at risk (i.e. on antiarrhythmic medications)

Aspirin (Ecotrin)

- Class: Antiplatelet, NSAID
- Mechanism of Action: Low dose aspirin inhibits thromboxane (an important factor that causes platelet aggregation); Inhibits Cyclooxygenase-1 and 2 (COX-1 and COX-2); results in a reduction in prostaglandins which cause pain, fever, inflammation
- Common Uses: Cardiovascular prophylaxis, pain, fever, inflammation
- Memorable Side Effects: GI ulcer, bleeding, worsening kidney function, edema, hypertension
- Clinical Pearls:
  - Rarely see aspirin used for pain or headache (primary use is cardiovascular prophylaxis – prevent stroke/heart attack)
  - Low dose aspirin is usually pretty well tolerated other than GI upset/bleed risk
  - NSAIDs are one of the most common causes of GI bleeding; this risk increases in the elderly and those on medications that increase risk of bleeding (anticoagulants and antiplatelet medications)
  - Because of the side effects of GI upset, NSAIDs should be taken with food (low dose aspirin usually ok without)
  - Due to effects on platelets, NSAIDs are typically held for a period of time before/after surgery to reduce the risk of bleeding
  - NSAIDs can contribute to edema and exacerbate CHF (congestive heart failure); be on the lookout and have NSAIDs reassessed if you see a patient with a CHF exacerbation or a patient requiring increasing diuretics like furosemide (usually not an issue with low dose aspirin)

Atenolol (Tenormin)

- Class: Beta-blocker, Antihypertensive
- Mechanism of Action: blocks beta receptors (aka beta-blocker)
- Common Uses: Atrial Fibrillation, hypertension
- Memorable Side Effects: low blood pressure and pulse, lethargy (sometimes patients can get used to this one)
- Clinical Pearls:
  - Trick to remembering beta receptors: You have 1 heart and 2 lungs (beta-1 is primarily on the heart and beta-2 primarily in the lungs). You will see beta receptors again with respiratory medications. If beta-1 is stimulated, heart rate increases. If beta-1 is blocked, heart rate decreases.
  - Atenolol is relatively selective for beta-1 only
  - Usually only dosed once daily which is a nice advantage over some other beta-blockers
  - Often in practice, providers will place a hold order on beta-blockers if the pulse is too low. This is obviously done to reduce the risk of significant bradycardia. Clinically it may depend upon the situation, but in an ambulatory setting, you may see the order set to hold the beta blocker when pulse is less than 55 or 60.

Atomoxetine (Strattera)

- Class: Norepinephrine reuptake inhibitor
- Mechanism of Action: Inhibits reuptake of norepinephrine
- Common Uses: ADHD
- Memorable Side Effects: sweating, dry mouth, GI, increase BP, weight loss
- Clinical Pearls:
  - Non-controlled substance used for ADHD is the big advantage of atomoxetine compared to methylphenidate, amphetamine salts, etc.
  - Special warning regarding increased risk of suicidal thoughts and behaviors
  - Can increase BP, cardiovascular problems, and increase risk of poor appetite/weight loss just like tradition stimulants (methylphenidate)

Atorvastatin (Lipitor)

- Class: Statin, Antilipemic
- Mechanism of Action: HMG Co-A reductase inhibitor (causes decrease in LDL)
- Common Uses: Reduction of cholesterol (particularly LDL)
- Memorable Side Effects: muscle aches, rhabdomyolysis (rare but serious)
- Clinical Pearls:
  - Statins like atorvastatin are one of the mainstays of therapy to reduce cholesterol, and more particularly LDL (bad cholesterol)
  - The most notable side effect with statins that you will likely hear patients complain about is myopathy (muscle aches/pain)
  - Usually muscle aches are all over which can help you differentiate from other pain conditions or pain/soreness from an injury or overuse
  - Contraindicated in pregnancy
  - Patients who do not tolerate atorvastatin, may try another statin as long as adverse effects aren't too severe (i.e. rhabdomyolysis); if you notice that the patient had an allergy or intolerance, you need to clarify with the provider
  - CPK will be the primary lab to test for rhabdomyolysis — breakdown of muscle; this elevation in CPK may eventually lead to kidney failure
  - If they are going to, patients usually will present with myopathy when the medication is first started or increased, but be on the lookout for new medications that can interact with statins like CYP3A4 inhibitor drug interactions with medications like fluconazole or erythromycin (this will cause

atorvastatin concentrations in the body to go up potentially leading to toxicity)
- o Gemfibrozil is a cholesterol medication that also interacts with atorvastatin – this drug interaction should be addressed with the primary provider
- o For many statins it is "recommended" to give them at night – the theory is cholesterol production happens at night

Atropine

- Class: Anticholinergic
- Mechanism of Action: Blocks acetylcholine in the parasympathetic system which decreases secretions and increases cardiac output
- Common Uses: Reduce salivary secretions; Pre-op as well as end of life, bradycardia
- Memorable Side Effects: Highly anticholinergic (can't spit, see, pee, poop)
- Clinical Pearls:
  - Oral drops used frequently in hospice to decrease excessive salivation
  - Can cause significant urinary retention
  - Psychotic type symptoms are possible with high enough doses ("mad as a hatter")
  - Pulse monitoring important (can cause tachycardia)
  - EKG monitoring critical if using for bradycardia

Azithromycin (Zithromax, Z-Pak)

- Class: Antibiotic, Macrolide
- Mechanism of Action: Inhibits protein synthesis in bacteria (macrolide class of antibiotics)
- Common Uses: Upper respiratory infections (i.e. ear infection, pneumonia, bronchitis, sinusitis)
- Memorable Side Effects: GI most common; QTc prolongation possible (very rare)
- Clinical Pearls:
  - Common alternative to amoxicillin (penicillin allergy is fairly common) in pediatrics or adults for that matter with bacterial ear infection, bronchitis, etc.
  - Really nice/easy dosing as azithromycin has a long half-life (classic Z-Pak is 2 tablets the first day then 1 tablet daily for the next four days) versus amoxicillin which needs to be dosed multiple times per day
  - Keep an eye out for patients with a history of arrhythmias or on medication for arrhythmias (amiodarone etc.) as azithromycin can potentially contribute to QTc prolongation
  - Much less likely to cause drug interactions compared to other macrolides like erythromycin and clarithromycin
  - Keep oral suspension (liquid formulation) at room temp!!! This is unique from many other liquids which are normally refrigerated

Baclofen (Lioresal)

- Class: Muscle relaxant
- Mechanism of Action: Acts in the CNS and produces muscle relaxation
- Common Uses: Muscle spasms
- Memorable Side Effects: Anticholinergic activity, sedation, fall risk, confusion
- Clinical Pearls:
  - One of the most common medications specifically for spasms (cyclobenzaprine is another classic example)
  - Will often see patients with multiple sclerosis struggle with spasms and on this medication
  - Anticholinergic side effects can be problematic, especially in the elderly
  - Sedation can increase fall risk
  - Can be given via pump (intrathecal)

Benazepril (Lotensin)

- Class: Antihypertensive, ACE Inhibitor
- Mechanism of Action: Benazepril inhibits the angiotensin converting enzyme. This prevents the production of angiotensin 2; less angiotensin 2 equates to less vasoconstriction, and lower blood pressure
- Common Uses: Hypertension, acute MI, heart failure
- Common Side Effects: Cough, kidney impairment, low blood pressure, and hyperkalemia
- Clinical Pearls:
  - ACE Inhibitors are notoriously known for causing a dry chronic cough
  - Angiotensin Receptor Blockers (ARBs) are the cousins to the ACE Inhibitors, and are the first line substitute to a patient who has had a cough with an ACE Inhibitor
  - ACE inhibitors can exacerbate kidney impairment as well as contribute to acute renal failure especially in patients who are already on other potential renal toxic medications (i.e. diuretics, NSAIDs etc.) even though in conditions like heart failure, diuretics and ACE Inhibitors are often used together
  - ACE Inhibitors are a classic cause of elevated potassium levels; if your patient has hyperkalemia, you must make sure the ACE Inhibitor has been addressed
  - In some cases, African Americans may not respond to ACE Inhibitors as well as other ethnicities
  - A common mistake I've seen clinicians make is using an ACE Inhibitor with an ARB; this is generally not recommended
  - ACE Inhibitors are frequently used in patients with hypertension and a history of diabetes, stroke, CAD, CKD, and CHF

Benzonatate (Tessalon)

- Class: Antitussive
- Mechanism of Action: Anesthetic effects on respiratory tract resulting in cough suppression
- Common Uses: Antitussive (cough)
- Memorable Side Effects: Usually pretty well tolerated, GI/possible CNS effects (rare)
- Clinical Pearls:
  - Very important to identify why patient is coughing
  - If coughing has been going on a long time be sure patients get assessed
  - ACE Inhibitors are classic cause of drug induced cough
  - An atypical cause of cough that won't resolve is heartburn or GERD (especially in elderly or young)
  - Asthma is another potential cause of chronic cough

Knowing the facts is one thing, learning how to apply your skills is the real challenge! Check out my #1 Amazon Best Seller which is packed full of my favorite medication cases and stories from the blog!

Benztropine (Cogentin)

- Class: Anticholinergic, Anti-Parkinson's agent
- Mechanism of Action: Blocks muscarinic (anticholinergic) receptors and also has antihistamine effects
- Common Uses: EPS associated with antipsychotic medications, Parkinsonism
- Memorable Side Effects: Anticholinergic, sedation
- Clinical Pearls:
  - Highly anticholinergic (can't spit, see, pee, or sh*t and confusion/fall risk)
  - Rarely used for Parkinson's because of the anticholinergic impacts in the elderly
  - Most often I've seen used for extrapyramidal disorders (movement side effects with antipsychotics)

Bisacodyl (Dulcolax)

- Class: Stimulant laxative
- Mechanism of Action: Stimulates GI movement by irritating smooth muscle
- Common Uses: Constipation
- Memorable Side Effects: Abdominal pain
- Clinical Pearls:
  - Used to promote bowel movement
  - Similar medication class as Sennosides
  - Suppository formulation is nice for patients who may have difficulty swallowing/can't take oral
  - Can be used as needed
  - Often used in treatment/prevention of opioid induced constipation

Bisoprolol (Zebeta)

- Class: Antihypertensive, Beta-blocker
- Mechanism of Action: Blocks beta receptors leading to lower pulse/BP
- Common Uses: Hypertension, Atrial fibrillation
- Memorable Side Effects: Low pulse, low BP, fatigue
- Clinical Pearls:
  - Trick to remembering beta receptors: You have 1 heart and 2 lungs (beta-1 is primarily on the heart and beta-2 primarily in the lungs)
  - If beta-1 is stimulated, heart rate increases. If beta-1 is blocked, heart rate decreases.
  - Bisoprolol is relatively selective for beta-1 only
  - Often in practice, providers will place a hold order on beta-blockers if the pulse is too low. This is obviously done to reduce the risk of significant bradycardia. Clinically it may depend upon the situation, but in an ambulatory setting, you may see the order set to hold the beta blocker when pulse is less than 55 or 60.

Budesonide – oral (Entocort)

- Class: Corticosteroid
- Mechanism of Action: Suppresses leukocytes and ultimately reduces inflammation, suppresses adrenal function and the immune system
- Common Uses: Acute inflammatory states (dermatitis, arthritis flare, Crohn's, pneumonia, asthma exacerbation, etc.)
- Memorable Side Effects: GI side effects, insomnia, hyperglycemia, long term use; suppress immune system, increase osteoporosis risk as well as cause adrenal insufficiency
- Clinical Pearls:
  o Budesonide is usually specifically reserved for ulcerative colitis or Crohn's disease
  o Be sure to take steroids with food as they can be pretty hard on the GI tract
  o In patients with diabetes, educate them that a fluctuation in blood sugars may occur when starting, changing doses, or discontinuing this medication due to the adverse effect of hyperglycemia
  o Long term corticosteroid use can lead to increased risk Cushing's (moon face), diabetes, and osteoporosis; make sure long term use is assessed frequently to minimize length and dose of steroids
  o In patients on long term use, they should be assessed if vitamin D and/or calcium and bisphosphonates should be added to reduce osteoporosis risk
  o Insomnia is common in the short term, but may resolve as short term use goes to longer term use

- o Short "bursts" 3 days to a week or 2 are often used to relieve acute inflammatory states causing patient distress (asthma, rheumatoid arthritis, etc.)
- o Corticosteroids (especially long term and higher doses) can also suppress the immune system
- o Is also available as a nebulized inhaled corticosteroid (brand name – Pulmicort) for asthma/COPD/respiratory issues

Bupropion (Wellbutrin, Zyban)

- Class: Antidepressant (non-SSRI)
- Mechanism of Action: Not well understood, thought to increase dopamine/norepinephrine (NOT serotonin)
- Common Uses: Depression, smoking cessation
- Memorable Side Effects: Insomnia/activating, increases seizure risk, GI side effects
- Clinical Pearls:
  - Generally not used first line for depression unless a patient is also looking to stop smoking
  - Tends to be more activating (insomnia adverse effect)
  - Less risk of reduced libido compared to SSRI's
  - Avoid if possible in a patient with a seizure history

Buspirone (Buspar)

- Class: Anti-anxiety
- Mechanism of Action: Not well known, possible effects on serotonin, dopamine
- Common Uses: Anxiety
- Memorable Side Effects: Sedation (pretty well tolerated in the elderly compared to other anti-anxiety medications)
- Clinical Pearls:
  - Usually a much safer choice for treatment of anxiety versus benzodiazepines (especially elderly)
  - Big disadvantage is they take a while (weeks to months) to show benefit for anxiety
  - They don't work on an as needed basis
  - Not a controlled substance in the U.S. (benzodiazepines are)
  - Usually dosed multiple times per day

Calcium acetate (PhosLo)

- Class: Phosphate binder
- Mechanism of Action: Binds with dietary phosphate in the gut and gets excreted in the feces
- Common Uses: Hyperphosphatemia (Phosphate binder)
- Memorable Side Effects: Hypercalcemia, GI (N/V/D)
- Clinical Pearls:
  - Used as a phosphate binder usually in CKD as phosphate levels can build up in end stage renal disease
  - Dosed with meals
  - Need to watch calcium as this medication can increase levels

Carbamazepine (Tegretol)

- Class: Antiepileptic
- Mechanism of Action: Multiple mechanisms, including altering sodium ion flow across cell membranes
- Common Uses: Seizures, trigeminal neuralgia
- Memorable Side Effects: sedation, dizziness, rash, hyponatremia (SIADH), N/V
- Clinical Pearls:
  - Enzyme inducer, so can decrease concentrations of multiple other meds (drug interactions)
  - Liver Function, CBC, and sodium are important monitoring parameters
  - Lots of wacky side effects (rash, liver function, hyponatremia, CBC changes) with this medication
  - Levels likely not necessary for patients using this med for trigeminal neuralgia unless signs of toxicity
  - Sedation, confusion, falls are possible with toxicity
  - 4-12 mcg/mL is considered "normal" therapeutic concentration for seizures

Carbidopa/levodopa (Sinemet)

- Class: Anti-Parkinson's
- Mechanism of Action: Levodopa crosses the blood brain barrier and gets converted to dopamine; carbidopa prevents the peripheral breakdown of levodopa
- Common Uses: Parkinson's, restless leg syndrome
- Memorable Side Effects: Nausea/vomiting, hallucinations, orthostasis
- Clinical Pearls:
  - Levodopa replaces the body's dopamine supply (shortage of dopamine in Parkinson's)
  - Can cause psychotic type symptoms (remember that antipsychotics block dopamine)
  - GI upset/nausea is common
  - Frequent dosing (up to 6-8 times per day) may be necessary depending upon patient's symptoms
  - May see used at night for RLS

Carisoprodol (Soma)

- Class: Skeletal muscle relaxant
- Mechanism of Action: Not well understood, acts in the CNS and produces muscle relaxation
- Common Uses: Musculoskeletal pain
- Memorable Side Effects: Sedation, dizziness
- Clinical Pearls:
  - Controlled substance, so there is a risk of it being habit forming
  - Can cause cognitive changes, confusion, sedation etc. – higher risk in the elderly and also caution patients about driving
  - Generally used short term if possible
  - Rare – increased risk of lowering seizure threshold in patients with seizure disorder
  - Anticholinergic and sedative effects make skeletal muscle relaxants not well tolerated in the elderly

Carvedilol (Coreg)

- Class: Antihypertensive, Beta-blocker
- Mechanism of Action: Blocks beta receptors leading to lower pulse/BP (also has some alpha blocking activity which is different from most beta-blockers)
- Common Uses: Hypertension, Atrial fibrillation
- Memorable Side Effects: Low pulse, low BP, fatigue
- Clinical Pearls:
  - Trick to remembering beta receptors: You have 1 heart and 2 lungs (beta-1 is primarily on the heart and beta-2 primarily in the lungs)
  - Carvedilol has the additive effect of blocking alpha receptors compared to other beta-blockers
  - Often in practice, providers will place a hold order on beta-blockers if the pulse is too low; this is done to reduce the risk of significant bradycardia
  - Clinically it may depend upon the situation, but in an ambulatory setting, you may see the order set to hold the beta blocker when pulse is less than 55 or 60

Cefazolin (Ancef)

- Class: Cephalosporin, Antibiotic
- Mechanism of Action: Inhibits bacterial cell wall formation
- Common Uses: surgical prophylaxis, endocarditis (if bacteria sensitive), skin infections
- Memorable Side Effects: GI side effects most common, allergy, rash, seizure (rare)
- Clinical Pearls:
  - Cephalosporin antibiotic
  - Often used in surgery prophylaxis to prevent infections
  - Alternative to penicillin antibiotics (very low risk of cross reactivity, but is possible)
  - If using for treatment of an active infection, patients should begin improving within a couple days if drug is working

Cefdinir (Omnicef)

- Class: Cephalosporin, Antibiotic
- Mechanism of Action: Inhibits bacterial cell wall formation
- Common Uses: skin infections, ear infection, sinusitis, strep throat,
- Memorable Side Effects: GI side effects most common, allergy, rash
- Clinical Pearls:
  - Third generation cephalosporin
  - It is often used as an alternative to amoxicillin, however with its chemical structure, it is somewhat related to the penicillin's (cross reactivity risk is low)
  - As with most antibiotics, usual adverse effects are GI upset/diarrhea related
  - Usually dosed multiple times per day which can be an issue for patient adherence

Ceftriaxone (Rocephin)

- Class: Cephalosporin, Antibiotic
- Mechanism of Action: Inhibits bacterial cell wall formation
- Common Uses: pneumonia, gonorrhea, skin infections
- Memorable Side Effects: GI side effects, rash, changes in platelets, WBC's (rare)
- Clinical Pearls:
  - Very commonly used in pneumonia
  - Can be given IM as well as IV
  - Not contraindicated with penicillin allergy, cross reactivity low, but need to at least be aware
  - Be more cautious if patient has allergy to another cephalosporin
  - With most antibiotics, symptoms should start to get better within 2-4 days

Cefuroxime (Ceftin, Zinacef)

- Class: Cephalosporin, Antibiotic
- Mechanism of Action: Inhibits bacterial cell wall formation
- Common Uses: skin infections, ear infection, sinusitis, strep throat,
- Memorable Side Effects: GI side effects most common, allergy, rash
- Clinical Pearls:
  - Common use is upper respiratory bacterial infection (sinusitis or ear infection)
  - Alternative to penicillin antibiotics (very low risk of cross reactivity, but is possible)
  - Oral or IV formulation available
  - Patients should begin improving within a couple days if drug is working/being taken appropriately
  - If suspension used, you must adequately shake to disperse the medication!
  - Can take with meals to ease GI upset risk

Celecoxib (Celebrex)

- Class: COX-2 Inhibitor, Analgesic
- Mechanism of Action: Inhibits Cyclooxygenase-2 preferentially (COX-2); results in a reduction in prostaglandins which cause pain, fever, inflammation
- Common Uses: Pain, inflammation
- Memorable Side Effects: GI ulcer (less than traditional NSAIDs), worsening kidney function, edema, hypertension, inhibits platelets (can exacerbate bleed risk)
- Clinical Pearls:
    - COX-2 inhibitors can cause GI bleed, but the risk is much less than traditional NSAIDs - risk increases in the elderly and those on medications that increase risk of bleeding (anticoagulants and antiplatelet medications)
    - COX-2 inhibitors can contribute to edema and exacerbate CHF (congestive heart failure); be on the lookout and have celecoxib reassessed if you see a patient with a CHF exacerbation or a patient requiring increasing diuretics like furosemide
    - Celecoxib can cause worsening kidney function (creatinine should be monitored); this risk can be greatly increased in patients on ACE Inhibitors or ARBs and/or diuretic type medications
    - When you think of celecoxib, think NSAID side effects with less GI risk
    - Boxed warning for increased risk of heart attack (MI) and stroke

Cephalexin (Keflex)

- Class: Cephalosporin, Antibiotic
- Mechanism of Action: Inhibits bacterial cell wall formation
- Common Uses: skin infections, ear infection, sinusitis, strep throat,
- Memorable Side Effects: GI side effects most common, allergy, rash
- Clinical Pearls:
  - Very common antibiotic used for skin infections, upper respiratory problems like strep throat, bronchitis, ear infection
  - It is often used as an alternative to amoxicillin, however with its chemical structure, it is somewhat related to the penicillin's (cross reactivity risk is low)
  - As with most antibiotics, usual adverse effects are GI upset/diarrhea related
  - Usually dosed multiple times per day which can be an issue for patient adherence
  - With or without food is ok

Cetirizine (Zyrtec)

- Class: Antihistamine
- Mechanism of Action: Blocks H1 receptors
- Common Uses: Allergic rhinitis, itching
- Memorable Side Effects: Sedation (much less than 1st generation antihistamines like diphenhydramine or hydroxyzine), mildly anticholinergic
- Clinical Pearls:
  - Second generation antihistamine (first generation example would be diphenhydramine)
  - Second generation H1 blockers like cetirizine are generally first line for seasonal allergies as they are more tolerable than first generation antihistamines
  - Generally less sedating and less anticholinergic effects than first generation
  - Remember that histamine 1 receptor blockers are generally called antihistamines, while histamine 2 receptor blockers are acid blockers used for GI issues (ranitidine, famotidine, etc.)
  - Often with antihistamines, if one doesn't work, patients may try another one from the same class (loratadine, fexofenadine, etc.)

Ciprofloxacin (Cipro)

- Class: Quinolone, Antibiotic
- Mechanism of Action: Inhibits bacterial DNA synthesis
- Common Uses: UTI's
- Memorable Side Effects: GI side effects, QTc prolongation (rare)
- Clinical Pearls:
  - Commonly used for the treatment of UTI's; great coverage against many gram negative bacteria
  - Dose adjustments might be necessary in patients with poor kidney function
  - Should not be co-administered with iron or calcium products as this can significant reduce absorption and possibly lead to treatment failure
  - Generally NOT used for pneumonia (Other quinolones like levofloxacin and moxifloxacin can be) – has poor activity against Strep. pneumoniae (a common cause of pneumonia)
  - Usually has to be dosed multiple times per day (at least twice)
  - Spontaneous tendon rupture has been reported with quinolones (extremely rare)

Citalopram (Celexa)

- Class: SSRI, Antidepressant
- Mechanism of Action: SSRI – selective serotonin reuptake inhibitor; increases serotonin in the brain
- Common Uses: Depression, anxiety, PTSD
- Memorable Side Effects: GI side effects (N/V/D), can really cause sedation or activation depending upon the patient, changes in mental status, hyponatremia (rare)
- Clinical Pearls:
  - The dose of citalopram should be limited/monitored closely in the elderly as well as patients on omeprazole
  - SSRI's are generally considered the first line medication to treat depression, they are generally well tolerated, and less risky than other antidepressants in the situation of suicide by overdosing on pills
  - Stomach/GI complaints/diarrhea are probably the most common SE's
  - There may be an increased risk of suicidal thinking when first starting these medications (there is a BOXED warning for this risk)
  - Although not terribly common, hyponatremia (low sodium) is a possible unique side effect with SSRI's and much more likely in patients already prone to hyponatremia – classic example would be patients who are taking diuretics, which can also lower sodium
  - Remember that these drugs are not an immediate fix! In most cases, SSRI's take weeks sometimes months before a patient will start improving; however side effects will be apparent from the start of the medication, making it difficult to coach our

patients to continue the medication in the first few weeks after starting it

- SSRI's are used in pregnancy, but the risk versus the benefit needs to be assessed on a case by case basis
- SSRI's can decrease libido

Clindamycin (Cleocin)

- Class: Antibiotic, Lincosamide
- Mechanism of Action: Inhibits bacterial protein synthesis
- Common Uses: Skin, bone, joint infections
- Memorable Side Effects: GI side effects, colitis (C. diff risk), metallic taste
- Clinical Pearls:
  - Has some activity again MRSA (methicillin resistant Staph. aureus) where penicillin antibiotics would not be effective
  - Possible alternative for patients who need antibiotic prophylaxis undergoing dental procedures who can't tolerate or have an allergy to penicillin antibiotics
  - One of the common antibiotics that may contribute to C. diff development (quinolones, cephalosporin's, and penicillin's may contribute as well)
  - Frequent administration is kind of a nuisance – usually 3-4 times per day
  - Recommended to give with a full glass of water to minimize esophageal ulceration risk

Clobetasol (Temovate)

- Class: Corticosteroid, Topical
- Mechanism of Action: Topical corticosteroid - Suppresses mediators of inflammation (histamine, kinins, prostaglandins etc.) resulting in less inflammation/redness
- Common Uses: Dermatitis
- Memorable Side Effects: local irritation - systemic side effects can happen but rare; prolonged use, large areas increase systemic absorption and risk of adrenal suppression, HPA-axis suppression, etc.
- Clinical Pearls:
  - If patients don't see improvement in condition in 1-2 weeks, be sure they know to get reassessed
  - Long term use (especially if large amounts/areas of the body can lead to significant systemic absorption) can suppress the HPA axis
  - Long term use probably more concerning in young children
  - Systemic problems not likely if used short term

Clonazepam (Klonopin)

- Class: Antianxiety, Benzodiazepine
- Mechanism of Action: enhances activity of GABA (an inhibitor neurotransmitter that causes sedation)
- Common Uses: Anxiety, insomnia
- Memorable Side Effects: sedation, confusion, fall risk, dizziness
- Clinical Pearls:
  - The best way I remember benzodiazepines is that they are very close to "alcohol in a pill"
  - Sedation, slurred speech, trouble walking (ataxia) etc. are all common with benzo's/alcohol; they are also commonly used in alcohol withdrawal
  - Be cautious with patients on higher doses of benzodiazepines to make sure they aren't abruptly stopped
  - Educate patients on driving/operating machinery (remember that benzodiazepines are often used for sleep as well as anxiety
  - Unlike SSRI's for anxiety, a great advantage of benzo's are that they work quickly and can be used as needed
  - Falls in the elderly is a big downside to using these medications
  - Benzo's are a controlled substance, i.e. they can cause addiction etc.
  - Flumazenil is antidote in overdose

Clonidine (Catapres)

- Class: Antihypertensive, Alpha-2 agonist
- Mechanism of Action: Centrally acting alpha-2 agonist which results in decreased sympathetic activity and drop in blood pressure
- Common Uses: Hypertension, psych issues like ADHD
- Memorable Side Effects: Drowsiness, dizziness, dry mouth
- Clinical Pearls:
  - Not the best in the elderly (on Beer's list)
  - Mainly used in hypertension, but occasionally will see it used off label for various psych issues
  - Comes in a patch formulation (and oral tabs) which may be advantageous for patients who can't swallow, take pills, etc.
  - Low BP and Pulse is possible
  - Sedating which can be a significant problem especially in the elderly

Clopidogrel (Plavix)

- Class: Antiplatelet, Thienopyridine
- Mechanism of Action: Blocks ADP receptors (leads to inhibition of platelets)
- Common Uses: MI, Stroke prevention
- Memorable Side Effects: Bleeding (GI, nose bleeds etc.)
- Clinical Pearls:
  - Clopidogrel is often used after a heart attack (MI) with aspirin to prevent further heart attacks; how long a patient should remain on this medication can vary depending upon cardiac and/or stroke risk – length of therapy should be addressed by the primary provider and in many situations may be 12 months, but can be longer or indefinite depending upon risk factors
  - Clopidogrel is a substitute if a patient cannot take or tolerate aspirin to help prevent stroke or heart attack
  - Due to its ability to inhibit platelets, the major complication is bleeding – assess patients for bruising, blood in the stool, any abnormal sign of bleeding etc.
  - CBC (hemoglobin and platelets in particular) are going to be one of the most important labs to monitor

Codeine / APAP (Tylenol #3)

- Class: Analgesic, Opioid, (see acetaminophen)
- Mechanism of Action: Binds opioid receptors inhibiting CNS pain pathways and causes pain relief; acetaminophen is believed to inhibit prostaglandin production, but does not have anti-inflammatory effects like NSAIDs
- Common Uses: Management of pain disorders, both chronic and acute
- Memorable Side Effects: Constipation, sedation, respiratory depression, CNS effects like confusion, delirium etc., liver toxicity (acetaminophen in large doses >4 grams/day)
- Clinical Pearls:
  - Codeine is actually a prodrug of morphine; when it enters the body, it gets metabolized to morphine which has opioid activity and is primarily responsible for pain relief
  - With opioids we need to remember that prevention of constipation is important
  - Another combination product with acetaminophen, need to educate/monitor patients for use of other medications that contain acetaminophen
  - Sedation and CNS effects are often problematic with opioids
  - Driving/working machinery is certainly risky when using opioids as they can cause significant sedation (usually patients get used to this side effect if they take the medication chronically)
  - Codeine with acetaminophen is a schedule 3 controlled substance

Colchicine (Colcrys)

- Class: Anti-gout agent
- Mechanism of Action: inhibits Beta-tubulin ultimately inhibiting action of neutrophils that may contribute to gout symptoms
- Common Uses: Gout
- Memorable Side Effects: Diarrhea, nausea
- Clinical Pearls:
  - Diarrhea very prominent side effect
  - Cleared by the kidney, so may need to use lower doses in CKD
  - Can be used for acute gout flare or prophylaxis (unique from allopurinol which is only used for prophylaxis of gout)
  - Always be on the lookout for medications that can elevate uric acid when you see an Rx for colchicine like thiazide diuretics, niacin etc.

Conjugated Estrogen (Premarin)

- Class: Estrogen Derivative
- Mechanism of Action: Mimics body's natural estrogen
- Common Uses: Menopausal symptoms, osteoporosis, uterine bleeding, vaginal atrophy (due to menopause)
- Memorable Side Effects: GI side effects, clot formation (DVT/PE), increased risk of certain types of cancers (endometrial and breast)
- Clinical Pearls:
  - Most often used for estrogen replacement in postmenopausal women
  - Alleviates troublesome hot flashes
  - Big risk is increase in certain types of cancer as well as clot formation (DVT); long term use is not recommended if possible
  - Positive bone effects (good in patients with osteoporosis)

Cyclobenzaprine (Flexeril)

- Class: Skeletal Muscle Relaxant
- Mechanism of Action: Acts in the CNS and produces muscle relaxation
- Common Uses: Muscle spasms
- Memorable Side Effects: Anticholinergic activity, sedation, fall risk, confusion
- Clinical Pearls:
  - Normally used to relax the muscles in the case of muscle spasms, hopefully this medication only needs to be used for a short period of time
  - Elderly may particularly be at risk for side effects like anticholinergic effects, sedation, dizziness (fall risk)
  - Onset of action is pretty quick (around an hour) so this medication can be used on an as needed basis
  - With the sedation side effect, we always need to caution our patients about driving, using machinery, etc.
  - Dry mouth is common especially with frequent use

Dabigatran (Pradaxa)

- Class: Anticoagulant, Thrombin inhibitor
- Mechanism of Action: Direct thrombin inhibitor which leads to prevention of blood clots
- Common Uses: Atrial fibrillation, DVT
- Memorable Side Effects: Bleeding
- Clinical Pearls:
  - Bleed risk! Monitor for bruising, low hemoglobin, blood in stools, nose bleeds etc.
  - GI bleed risk is especially problematic when used with NSAIDs (ibuprofen, naproxen, etc.)
  - There is a reversal agent available! (expensive)
  - Twice daily dosing makes it a little inconvenient
  - Be aware to have provider assess for dose adjustment in patients with CKD
  - Alternative to warfarin and routine INR is not necessary

Darbepoetin alfa (Aranesp)

- Class: Erythropoiesis Stimulating Agent (ESA)
- Mechanism of Action: Stimulates the production of red blood cells (mimics the body's natural erythropoietin which is produced by the kidney)
- Common Uses: Anemia from CKD, anemia from chemotherapy/cancer
- Memorable Side Effects: Hypertension, GI, Injection site reaction, increase clot risk (boxed warning)
- Clinical Pearls:
  o Lack of iron stores may inhibit response
  o Monitor hemoglobin/hematocrit for response (should increase)
  o Risk of hypertension
  o There should be hold parameters in place (i.e. hold if hemoglobin is greater than 11)
  o Longer acting form of erythropoietin (advantage is you don't have to give it as often)
  o Important boxed warning on increased risk of MI, stroke, blood clots

Dexlansoprazole (Dexilant)

- Class: Proton Pump Inhibitor
- Mechanism of Action: Inhibits proton pumps in the stomach leading to a less acidic environment
- Common Uses: GERD, ulcer, Barrett's esophagus
- Memorable Side Effects: Usually pretty well tolerated; Long term use: Possibility to increase fracture risk, decrease B12 levels, C. diff risk, low magnesium
- Clinical Pearls:
  - PPI's are the most potent acid blocker on the market
  - PPI's are generally dosed 30 minutes or so before meals – this is a recommendation, not an absolute (example if a patient likes to get up and eat right away upon rising, the medication will still likely be beneficial, but may not have a maximal effect)
  - For some patients PPI's may not work very quickly, i.e. it might take a few days for maximal effect
  - For the above reason, as needed (PRN) PPI's can possibly be effective, but are generally not used
  - Use short term if possible due to increased risk of osteoporosis, C. Diff, low magnesium, and B12 deficiency if used long term
  - Barrett's esophagus, high risk GI medications (i.e. NSAIDs, prednisone), or chronic GI bleed are examples where patients may require indefinite therapy
  - If GI bleed is problematic, monitoring hemoglobin and/or hemoccult (blood in the stool) might be appropriate to assess possible blood loss

Dexmethylphenidate (Focalin)

- Class: CNS Stimulant
- Mechanism of Action: Blocks reuptake of norepinephrine and dopamine leading to CNS stimulation (by blocking reuptake, you end up with more norepinephrine and dopamine in the synapse leading to more activity)
- Common Uses: ADHD, depression/fatigue (off label)
- Memorable Side Effects: Anxiety, insomnia, poor appetite, weight loss, hypertension, pulse, emotional lability
- Clinical Pearls:
  - Remembering that this medication ramps you up (stimulant) will help you remember its side effects (anxiety, insomnia, weight loss, poor appetite, increased BP, increased pulse etc.)
  - When used in pediatrics, poor appetite can be a significant problem and should be something that should be assessed
  - Elevated BP and pulse monitoring important
  - Be cautious in adult patients who may have cardiovascular risk (hypertension etc.)
  - Schedule 2 controlled substance, highly addictive

Diazepam (Valium)

- Class: Antianxiety, Antiepileptic
- Mechanism of Action: enhances activity of GABA (an inhibitor neurotransmitter that causes sedation)
- Common Uses: Anxiety, muscle spasms, seizures, insomnia
- Memorable Side Effects: sedation, confusion, fall risk, dizziness
- Clinical Pearls:
  - The best way I remember benzodiazepines is that they are very close to "alcohol in a pill"
  - Diazepam specifically has a long half-life in the elderly, so significant potential for accumulation of the drug exists when used in the elderly
  - Sedation, slurred speech, trouble walking (ataxia) etc. are all common with benzo's/alcohol; they are also commonly used in alcohol withdrawal
  - Be cautious with patients on higher doses of benzodiazepines to make sure they aren't abruptly stopped
  - Educate patients on driving/operating machinery (remember that benzodiazepines are often used for sleep as well as anxiety)
  - Unlike SSRI's for anxiety, a great advantage of benzo's are that they work quickly and can be used as needed
  - Falls in the elderly is a big downside to using these medications
  - Benzo's are a controlled substance, i.e. they can cause addiction etc.
  - Rectal/injectable formulation can be used in acute treatment of seizures
  - Flumazenil is antidote in overdose

Dicyclomine (Bentyl)

- Class: GI Antispasmodic, Anticholinergic
- Mechanism of Action: Blocks acetylcholine receptors (anticholinergic)
- Common Uses: Irritable bowel syndrome
- Memorable Side Effects: Anticholinergic effects (can't spit, see, pee or poop)
- Clinical Pearls:
  - Primary use is to help relieve GI spasms/pain due to irritable bowel syndrome
  - Anticholinergic (so will slow the GI tract and decrease spasms) side effects can be prominent especially in the elderly population
  - Usually dosed multiple times throughout the day
  - If diarrhea is an issue associated with a patient's IBS, the anticholinergic effect of constipation can certainly contribute to the patient's benefit

Digoxin (Digitek, Lanoxin)

- Class: Antiarrhythmic, Cardiac Glycoside
- Mechanism of Action: Inhibition of sodium/potassium ATPase
- Common Uses: Atrial fibrillation, heart failure
- Memorable Side Effects: nausea, vomiting, bradycardia, cognitive changes, weight loss, visual changes (usually at very high levels)
- Clinical Pearls:
  - Classic symptoms of digoxin toxicity involve GI side effects, bradycardia, cognitive changes and weight loss
  - Often providers will use hold parameters in healthcare settings to prevent pulse from going to low (i.e. hold digoxin if pulse is less than 60)
  - Digoxin is cleared by the kidney; it can accumulate and be much more likely to cause toxicity in the elderly as patients tend to have worse kidney function as they age
  - Higher doses are usually used in atrial fibrillation as compared to heart failure
  - Upper limit of normal for a digoxin level is considered 2 ng/mL
  - Patients with low levels of potassium are at greater risk of toxicity, it is really important to assess potassium as many patients on digoxin may also be on diuretics (usually for heart failure) that can deplete potassium

Diltiazem (Cardizem CD, Cartia XT)

- Class: Calcium Channel Blocker (non-dihydropyridine), antiarrhythmic
- Mechanism of Action: Blocks calcium channels resulting in vasodilation and cardiac relaxation
- Common Uses: Atrial fibrillation, hypertension
- Memorable Side Effects: Low pulse, low BP, constipation, edema
- Clinical Pearls:
  - Very important distinction: Verapamil and Diltiazem (non-dihydropyridine's) are the calcium channel blockers that act on the heart AND blood vessels; you will not see amlodipine and nifedipine used in atrial fibrillation, because their activity is primarily on the vessels. This also means that pulse monitoring will not be necessary with nifedipine and amlodipine
  - The higher you push the dose on these medications, the more likely you will see the side effect of edema; keep an eye out for new diuretic Rx's to treat the edema caused by the calcium channel blockers
  - Simvastatin is a very common medication that interacts with diltiazem
  - Comes in several different formulations (long acting, short acting etc.), make sure you have the right one

Diphenoxylate/atropine (Lomotil)

- Class: Antidiarrheal
- Mechanism of Action: Diphenoxylate inhibits GI motility (atropine is highly anticholinergic)
- Common Uses: Treatment of diarrhea
- Memorable Side Effects: Pretty well tolerated - Abdominal distress, possibility of anticholinergic effects, but not very likely as atropine dose is very low
- Clinical Pearls:
  - Controlled substance
  - Can be used as needed
  - Be sure patients who are on this chronically have been assessed for medical and possible medication concerns for chronic diarrhea

Divalproex (Valproic Acid, Depakote)

- Class: Antiepileptic, Mood stabilizer
- Mechanism of Action: Increases GABA (inhibitory neurotransmitter)
- Common Uses: Seizures, bipolar disorder, migraine prophylaxis
- Memorable Side Effects: CNS (sedation, dizziness), GI (N/V/stomach pain), hair loss – lots of rare side effects: possible effects on platelets, ammonia levels, LFTs etc.
- Clinical Pearls:
  - Checking drug levels usually not as important when using for mood or headaches (compared to seizures) unless trying to rule out toxicity
  - Frequent dosing - 2 or 3 times per day
  - Critical to ensure patients are taking! (Especially for seizures)
  - If using for seizures, be sure to have patient assess for meds that lower seizure threshold (bupropion, tramadol are classic examples)
  - Does have some drug interactions (i.e. lamotrigine)
  - Pregnancy category X for Migraines

Donepezil (Aricept)

- Class: Dementia agent, Acetylcholinesterase inhibitor
- Mechanism of Action: Inhibits acetylcholinesterase which increases acetylcholine in the CNS
- Common Uses: Alzheimer's dementia
- Memorable Side Effects: GI (N/V/D), weight loss, insomnia
- Clinical Pearls:
  - One of the more common drug causes of weight loss in the elderly
  - Usually dosed at night (to minimize GI risk, but rarely can cause insomnia)
  - Likely will NOT reverse dementia symptoms, but used to delay progression (prevent patients from getting worse)
  - Dementia medications in general can contribute to behavioral changes (good or bad)

Dopamine

- Class: Adrenergic agonist
- Mechanism of Action: Stimulates adrenergic and dopamine receptors
- Common Uses: shock, heart failure
- Memorable Side Effects: BP, Pulse changes, N/V, arrhythmia
- Clinical Pearls:
  - At low doses may actually cause renal vasodilation
  - At higher doses more likely to act like epinephrine (stimulates heart and vasoconstriction – increase pulse/BP)
  - Usually volume replacement is first in kidney failure, but this may be used adjunct in certain situations for shock

Doxazosin (Cardura)

- Class: Alpha blocker, Antihypertensive
- Mechanism of Action: Blocks alpha receptors causing smooth muscle relaxation, vasodilation and opening of the ureter
- Common Uses: BPH, urinary obstruction, hypertension
- Memorable Side Effects: Low BP, dizziness
- Clinical Pearls:
  - Non-selective alpha blocker, so can be used for both hypertension and BPH
  - Risk of orthostasis higher with a non-selective alpha blocker
  - In the case of worsening urinary retention due to BPH and initiation of these agents, be sure to assess if your patient is on anticholinergic medications (diphenhydramine, TCA's etc.)
  - Usually dosed at night to minimize the risk of orthostasis

Doxycycline (Vibramycin)

- Class: Tetracycline, Antibiotic
- Mechanism of Action: Inhibits bacterial protein synthesis
- Common Uses: Often an alternative to penicillin antibiotics (skin infections, pneumonia, etc.)
- Memorable Side Effects: GI side effects, photosensitivity (increased risk of sunburn), rash
- Clinical Pearls:
  - May give with meals if GI upset is a problem
  - Can cause birth defects (category D)
  - It is from the tetracycline class, so if patients have a tetracycline allergy, it shouldn't be used
  - Can make patients more susceptible to sunburn
  - Possibility to cause tooth discoloration (usually long term use only or multiple courses)
  - Avoid timing calcium, iron, antacids at the same time (may block absorption and decrease amount of drug absorbed)

Duloxetine (Cymbalta)

- Class: SNRI, Antidepressant
- Mechanism of Action: Selective serotonin and norepinephrine reuptake inhibitor (SNRI)
- Common Uses: Depression, pain syndromes (neuropathy especially), fibromyalgia
- Memorable Side Effects: GI side effects, can exacerbate hypertension (usually only at higher doses), CNS changes
- Clinical Pearls:
  - Has effects on both serotonin and norepinephrine
  - Duloxetine is indicated to help with pain syndromes as well depression; neuropathic pain in particular is where you will likely see it used most frequently
  - GI and central nervous system side effects (CNS) will likely be the most common
  - Decreased libido can be an issue for patients taking duloxetine
  - Be careful with the risk of serotonin syndrome especially in patients on other serotonergic medications

Dutasteride (Avodart)

- Class: 5-apha reductase inhibitor
- Mechanism of Action: Inhibits 5-alpha reductase which results in less dihydrotestosterone
- Common Uses: BPH
- Memorable Side Effects: Impotence, weakness
- Clinical Pearls:
  - Not for immediate relief of acute urinary retention due to BPH!
  - Takes weeks to months for clinical benefit
  - Pretty well tolerated usually with impotence being most common
  - Keep an eye out for drugs that exacerbate BPH (anticholinergics)

Enalapril (Vasotec)

- Class: Antihypertensive, ACE Inhibitor
- Mechanism of Action: Enalapril inhibits the angiotensin converting enzyme which prevents the production of angiotensin 2. Angiotensin 2 is a potent vasoconstrictor - Less angiotensin 2 equates to less vasoconstriction, and lower blood pressure
- Common Uses: Hypertension, acute MI, heart failure
- Common Side Effects: Cough, kidney impairment, low blood pressure, and hyperkalemia
- Clinical Pearls:
  - ACE Inhibitors are notoriously known for causing a dry chronic cough
  - If you ever have a patient with a chronic cough, you must assess if they are on an ACE Inhibitor.
  - Angiotensin Receptor Blockers (ARBs) are the cousins to the ACE Inhibitors, and are the first line substitute to a patient who has had a cough with an ACE Inhibitor
  - ACE inhibitors can exacerbate kidney impairment as well as contribute to acute renal failure especially in patients who are already on other potential renal toxic medications (i.e. diuretics, NSAIDs etc.) even though in conditions like heart failure, diuretics and ACE Inhibitors are often used together
  - ACE Inhibitors are a classic cause of elevated potassium levels; if your patient has hyperkalemia, you must make sure the ACE Inhibitor has been addressed
  - In some cases, African Americans may not respond to ACE Inhibitors as well as other ethnicities
  - A mistake I've seen clinicians make is using an ACE Inhibitor with and ARB; this is generally not recommended

- ACE Inhibitors (and ARBs) are frequently used in patients with hypertension and a history of diabetes, stroke, CAD, CKD, and CHF
- Angioedema (swelling of the lips/airway) is classically caused by ACE inhibition; it is extremely rare, but very serious requiring immediate discontinuation

Enoxaparin (Lovenox)

- Class: Anticoagulant, Low Molecular Weight Heparin
- Mechanism of Action: Primarily inhibits factor 10A clotting factor (anticoagulant)
- Common Uses: Used in MI, DVT prophylaxis, DVT treatment
- Memorable Side Effects: Bleed risk
- Clinical Pearls:
  - Bleeding risk is the major adverse effect that needs to be monitored with any medication that inhibits clotting factors
  - It is a heparin based product (low molecular weight heparin) so risk of heparin induced thrombocytopenia is there, but much lower than heparin
  - Checking INR's with Enoxaparin is not necessary; weight based dosing
  - Platelets and Hemoglobin are two important monitoring parameters (part of a CBC)
  - Often patients are bridged to warfarin with orders to start warfarin, and follow INR and when INR is 2 or greater, then discontinue enoxaparin
  - Significantly higher dose of enoxaparin recommended for treatment of blood clot (DVT) versus prevention
  - Injection only is a downside and why patients are often transitioned to an oral anticoagulant

Epinephrine (EpiPen, Adrenalin)

- Class: Alpha and Beta Agonist
- Mechanism of Action: Stimulates alpha and beta receptors
- Common Uses: Treatment of anaphylactic reactions, hypotension/shock
- Memorable Side Effects: tachycardia, hypertension, anxiety, insomnia, dry mouth, urinary retention
- Clinical Pearls:
  o Ramps you up! (Increase in BP, pulse, anxiety, irritability etc.)
  o Drug found in "Epi-pen" for severe allergic reactions
  o Epinephrine is used in the ACLS algorithm as well

Erythromycin (Ery-tab)

- Class: Macrolide, Antibiotic
- Mechanism of Action: Inhibits protein synthesis in bacteria (macrolide class of antibiotics)
- Common Uses: Upper respiratory i.e. ear infection, pneumonia, bronchitis, sinusitis; also used chronically for gastroparesis
- Memorable Side Effects: GI most common; QTc prolongation possible (very rare)
- Clinical Pearls:
  - Numerous drug interactions (compared to azithromycin), rarely used as an antibiotic due to this reason
  - Dosed multiple times per day (azithromycin much simpler dosing)
  - If see used chronically at low doses, likely being used to improve gastroparesis (slow GI motility common with diabetes)

Erythropoietin (Procrit, Epogen)

- Class: Erythropoiesis Stimulating Agent (ESA)
- Mechanism of Action: Stimulates the production of red blood cells
- Common Uses: Anemia from CKD, anemia from chemotherapy/cancer
- Memorable Side Effects: Hypertension, GI, Injection site reaction, increase clot risk (boxed warning)
- Clinical Pearls:
  - Lack of iron may inhibit response
  - Monitor hemoglobin/hematocrit for response (should increase)
  - Risk of hypertension
  - There should be hold parameters in place (i.e. hold if hemoglobin is greater than 11)
  - Important boxed warning on increased risk of MI, stroke, blood clots

Escitalopram (Lexapro)

- Class: Antidepressant, SSRI
- Mechanism of Action: SSRI – selective serotonin reuptake inhibitor; increases serotonin in the brain
- Common Uses: Depression, anxiety, PTSD
- Memorable Side Effects: GI side effects (N/V/D), can really cause sedation or activation depending upon the patient, changes in mental status, hyponatremia (rare)
- Clinical Pearls:
  - SSRI's are generally considered the first line medication to treat depression, they are generally well tolerated, and less risky than other antidepressants in the situation of suicide attempt through overdosing on pills
  - Stomach/GI complaints like stomach upset and/or diarrhea are probably the most common complications
  - There may be an increased risk of suicidal thinking when first starting these medications (there is a BOXED warning for this risk)
  - Although not terribly common, hyponatremia (low sodium) is a possible unique side effect with SSRI's and much more likely in patients already prone to hyponatremia – classic example would be patients who are taking diuretics, which can also lower sodium
  - Remember that these drugs are not an immediate fix! In most cases, SSRI's take weeks sometimes months before a patient will start improving; however side effects will be apparent from the start of the medication, making it difficult to coach our patients to continue the medication in the first few weeks of therapy

- SSRI's are used in pregnancy, but the risk versus the benefits need to be assessed on a case by case basis
- SSRI's can decrease libido

Esomeprazole (Nexium)

- Class: Proton Pump Inhibitor (PPI)
- Mechanism of Action: Inhibits proton pumps in the stomach leading to a less acidic environment
- Common Uses: GERD, ulcer, Barrett's esophagus
- Memorable Side Effects: Usually pretty well tolerated; Long term use: Possibility to increase fracture risk, decrease B12 levels, C. diff risk, low magnesium
- Clinical Pearls:
  - PPI's are the most potent acid blocker on the market
  - PPI's are generally dosed 30 minutes or so before meals – this is a recommendation, not an absolute (example if a patient likes to get up and eat right away upon rising, the medication will still likely be beneficial, but may not have a maximal effect)
  - For some patients PPI's may not work very quickly, i.e. it might take a few days for maximal effect
  - For the above reason, as needed (PRN) PPI's can possibly be effective, but are generally not used
  - Use short term if possible due to increased risk of osteoporosis, low magnesium, and B12 deficiency if used long term
  - Most common primary outcome of PPI would be to improve symptoms likely heartburn and stomach from GERD, stomach ulcer, or other related conditions
  - Barrett's esophagus, high risk GI medications (i.e. NSAIDs, prednisone), or chronic GI bleed may require indefinite therapy
  - If GI bleed is problematic, monitoring hemoglobin and/or hemoccult might be appropriate to assess possible blood loss

Eszopiclone (Lunesta)

- Class: Sedative, "Z" Drug
- Mechanism of Action: enhances activity of GABA (an inhibitor neurotransmitter that causes sedation)
- Common Uses: Insomnia
- Memorable Side Effects: sedation, confusion, fall risk, dizziness, abnormal sleep behaviors (sleep walking, eating etc.)
- Clinical Pearls:
    - Often termed as a "Z" drug, medications like eszopiclone are sedating; when medications are sedating we always have to be mindful of the morning after and make sure patients realize that driving and/or operating machinery can be extremely dangerous
    - It is recommended to try to use these medications only for short term if possible
    - Non-drug interventions such as sleep hygiene are the preferred treatment for insomnia
    - Before this type of medication is prescribed, keep an eye out for patients who may be on stimulating type medications or medications that can contribute to insomnia and make sure that these are assessed prior to giving a sleep medication – classic examples: methylphenidate, prednisone, too much levothyroxine, etc.
    - Eszopiclone is a controlled substance in the U.S.; there is a risk of addiction/dependence
    - Very similar effects to benzodiazepines (example: lorazepam)
    - Can increase risk of falls in our elderly patients

Etanercept (Enbrel)

- Class: DMARD (antirheumatic), TNF blocker
- Mechanism of Action: Blocks tumor necrosis factor (TNF) – TNF plays a role in the inflammatory process
- Common Uses: rheumatoid arthritis, psoriasis/psoriatic arthritis
- Memorable Side Effects: Infection risk (suppresses immune system), injection site reaction
- Clinical Pearls:
  - Watch for frequent infections or serious (suppresses immune system)
  - Acts as a controller of inflammatory conditions, not immediate relief
  - Expensive!!!
  - Injection
  - Refrigerated; but may warm to room temp to make injection less painful

Ethinyl Estradiol and Norgestimate (Ortho Tri-Cyclen, Sprintec, etc.)

- Class: Birth Control, Contraceptive
- Mechanism of Action: Inhibits ovulation by changing gonadotropin, FSH, and luteinizing hormone release
- Common Uses: Contraception, Acne
- Memorable Side Effects: Abnormal vaginal bleeding, DVT, hypertension
- Clinical Pearls:
  - Age, Smoking can put patients at higher risk of clot
  - Can exacerbate hypertension
  - Adherence to regimen is very important to prevent unplanned pregnancy
  - Enzyme inducers like carbamazepine, phenytoin can possibly reduce effectiveness of birth control

Ezetimibe (Zetia)

- Class: Antilipemic
- Mechanism of Action: Inhibits intestinal absorption of cholesterol
- Common Uses: Elevated cholesterol, particularly LDL
- Memorable Side Effects: Overall usually well tolerated, low risk of diarrhea, myopathy (especially when used in combo with statins)
- Clinical Pearls:
  - May be used in combination with a statin
  - Pretty well tolerated when used alone, but not nearly as potent at reducing LDL as statins
  - Still fairly expensive at this time (and don't get that great of LDL reduction)
  - Can possibly increase risk of rhabdomyolysis when added to statin therapy, so need to watch out for muscle pain/soreness etc.
  - Once daily dosing is nice

Famotidine (Pepcid)

- Class: H2 blocker
- Mechanism of Action: Blocks histamine 2 receptors (H2 blocker) which results in reduced gastric acid secretion and a higher pH in the stomach
- Common Uses: GERD, heartburn, GI bleed
- Memorable Side Effects: Pretty well tolerated overall (watch out for CNS changes in elderly and/or patients with poor kidney function)
- Clinical Pearls:
  - H2 blockers are cleared by the kidney, so they can accumulate/require dose adjustments in CKD
  - Generally less effective at suppressing stomach acid than PPI's
  - Available over the counter, inexpensive
  - CNS effects likely more common in elderly, on higher doses, and in patients with kidney disease
  - Generally used before PPI's if something more than Tums (calcium carbonate) is needed in pregnancy

Febuxostat (Uloric)

- Class: Anti-gout, Xanthine oxidase inhibitor
- Mechanism of Action: Inhibits xanthine oxidase resulting in decreased production of uric acid
- Common Uses: Gout prophylaxis
- Memorable Side Effects: rash, GI, liver function abnormalities (rare)
- Clinical Pearls:
  - Alternative to allopurinol for controlling uric acid levels in gout
  - NOT for treatment of acute flare
  - Keep an eye out for meds that may exacerbate gout (thiazide diuretics are the classic example)
  - Expensive alternative to allopurinol at this time

Fentanyl (Duragesic)

- Class: Opioid, Analgesic
- Mechanism of Action: Binds opioid receptors inhibiting CNS pain pathways
- Common Uses: Management of pain disorders, both chronic (patches only for chronic pain) and acute
- Memorable Side Effects: Constipation, sedation, CNS effects like confusion, delirium etc., respiratory depression
- Clinical Pearls:
  - Fentanyl is a scheduled 2 controlled substance; risk of addiction, dependence etc.
  - It is critical to educate/assess patients for constipation if they are taking scheduled opioids like fentanyl
  - Fentanyl patches are not recommended in patients who have never received an opioid before (opioid naïve patients)
  - Naloxone is reversal agent for opioids
  - Patches should never be used as needed; onset of pain relief is slow – hours to days
  - In most cases, flushing fentanyl patches is appropriate (risk of pets, children getting them out of garbage and overdosing)
  - 25 mcg patch is equivalent to approximately 60 mg of oral morphine per day (they are very potent)

Ferrous Sulfate

- Class: Iron Supplement
- Mechanism of Action: Replaces body's iron stores
- Common Uses: Iron deficiency anemia
- Memorable Side Effects: Constipation, black stools, GI pain
- Clinical Pearls:
  - Iron deficiency anemia is the most common use for iron supplements
  - In patients with CKD, anemia may likely be due to kidney disease versus iron deficiency (erythropoietin is produced in the kidney)
  - Constipation and black stools can be troublesome for patients – key education point
  - May be given with vitamin C to increase absorption (sometimes have seen with orange juice)

Fexofenadine (Allegra)

- Class: Antihistamine (2nd generation)
- Mechanism of Action: Blocks Histamine - 1 receptors
- Common Uses: Allergic rhinitis, itching
- Memorable Side Effects: Sedation (much less than 1st generation antihistamines like diphenhydramine or hydroxyzine), mildly anticholinergic
- Clinical Pearls:
    - Fexofenadine is a newer generation antihistamine, so it will have less anticholinergic effects than older antihistamines like diphenhydramine
    - Generally fairly well tolerated and is available over the counter
    - Usually only needs to be dosed once daily which is an advantage over some of the older antihistamines as well

Filgrastim (Neupogen)

- Class: Colony Stimulating Factor (CSF)
- Mechanism of Action: Stimulates production of WBC's
- Common Uses: Prevention of neutropenia in chemo patients
- Memorable Side Effects: Ostealgia (bone pain), anaphylaxis (rare)
- Clinical Pearls:
  - Helps patients continue on chemotherapy by increasing white blood cells
  - Bone pain is common (remember that it stimulates bone marrow which resides inside the bones – source of pain)
  - CBC (white blood cell count is incredibly important to monitor for response to treatment)
  - Fever and signs of infection are also incredibly important to watch for in a patient on filgrastim

Finasteride (Proscar)

- Class: 5 alpha reductase inhibitor
- Mechanism of Action: Inhibits 5-alpha reductase which results in less dihydrotestosterone
- Common Uses: BPH, baldness
- Memorable Side Effects: Impotence, weakness
- Clinical Pearls:
  - Not for immediate relief of acute urinary retention
  - Takes weeks to months for clinical benefit
  - Pretty well tolerated usually with impotence being most common
  - Hair growth
  - Keep an eye out for drugs that exacerbate BPH (anticholinergics)

Fluconazole (Diflucan)

- Class: Antifungal, Azole
- Mechanism of Action: Ultimately inhibits formation in fungal cell membrane
- Common Uses: Fungal infections like candidiasis, Cryptococcus
- Memorable Side Effects: GI side effects most common, Liver failure (very rare) more likely with chronic use
- Clinical Pearls:
  - Classically used to treat yeast infections (Candidiasis) and many simple patients may only require one dose
  - Notorious cause of drug interactions via CYP3A4 inhibition – It can increase concentrations of statins, seizure medications, etc. (if you see patients started on this medication, be sure to look up possible drug interactions)
  - Fungal infections are much more common in patients who are immunocompromised (i.e. AIDS, patient on immunosuppressant medications, etc.)
  - Can potentially cause prolonged QTc intervals especially in patients on other medications that prolong the QTc
  - Liver toxicity is rare, but should be monitored for especially if patients are receiving chronic therapy

Fluoxetine (Prozac)

- Class: SSRI, Antidepressant
- Mechanism of Action: SSRI – selective serotonin reuptake inhibitor; increases serotonin in the brain
- Common Uses: Depression, anxiety, PTSD
- Memorable Side Effects: GI side effects (N/V/D), can really cause sedation or activation depending upon the patient, changes in mental status, hyponatremia (rare)
- Clinical Pearls:
  - SSRI's are generally considered the first line medication to treat depression, they are generally well tolerated, and less risky than other antidepressants in the situation of attempted suicide through overdosing on pills
  - There may be an increased risk of suicidal thinking when first starting these medications (there is a BOXED warning for this risk)
  - In most patients, fluoxetine tends to be a little more activating versus sedating
  - Although not terribly common, hyponatremia (low sodium) is a possible unique side effect with SSRI's and much more likely in patients already prone to hyponatremia - classic example would be patients who are taking diuretics, which can also lower sodium
  - Remember that these drugs are not an immediate fix! In most cases, SSRI's take weeks sometimes months before a patient will start improving; however side effects can be apparent from the start of the medication, making it difficult to coach our patients to continue the medication in the first few weeks after starting it
  - SSRI's are used in pregnancy, but the risk versus the benefits need to be assessed on a case by case basis

- SSRI's can decrease libido

Fluticasone (Flonase)

- Class: Nasal Corticosteroid
- Mechanism of Action: Nasal steroid that helps to reduce inflammation
- Common Uses: Allergies
- Memorable Side Effects: Pretty well tolerated, likely nasal irritation, possible nose bleeds if any
- Clinical Pearls:
  - Gently shake the product for nasal inhalation and you may need to prime the nasal delivery device if it is the first time using it
  - There is also an oral inhalation product that is used for asthma/COPD – (brand is Flovent)
  - Educate patients that it may not work right away, it may take a few hours or up to a day or two to start working (because of this, it may not be the ideal to use this as needed, but I've certainly seen it prescribed this way before)
  - It may only be necessary to use this medication seasonally based upon timing and duration of allergy symptoms
  - Be sure to educate patients to clean the tip of the nasal delivery device as it can get pretty nasty!

Folic Acid

- Class: Folic acid supplement
- Mechanism of Action: Replacement of dietary folic acid
- Common Uses: Pregnancy, patients on methotrexate or other meds that cause low folic acid levels, folic acid deficiency (anemia)
- Memorable Side Effects: GI upset if anything, but virtually no side effects, water soluble so won't accumulate
- Clinical Pearls:
  - Folic acid supplementation is recommended in pregnancy to minimize risk of neural tube defects
  - Folic acid is given with methotrexate
  - Deficiency can lead to anemia
  - Found in nearly all multivitamins
  - Sulfasalazine and Trimethoprim are two medications that can potentially cause folic acid deficiency

Furosemide (Lasix)

- Class: Loop Diuretic
- Mechanism of Action (MOA): Inhibit sodium and chloride reabsorption in the ascending "Loop" of Henle in the kidney
- Common Use: edema, hypertension, heart failure
- Memorable Side Effects: frequent urination, electrolyte depletion, low blood pressure, dehydration and renal impairment
- Clinical Pearls:
  - While furosemide can cause significant reductions in magnesium, calcium, sodium etc., potassium is one of the most important electrolytes to monitor and often patients require potassium supplementation; this can sometimes be offset by potassium sparing diuretics like spironolactone, ARBs like losartan, and ACE inhibitors like Lisinopril (all potentially increase potassium)
  - Frequent urination can be significantly upsetting to patients and can greatly impact their wellbeing, including upsetting their sleep; make sure these loop diuretics are not being given too close to bedtime (if possible) and waking up our patients
  - Whenever you see a new Rx for a loop diuretic, be sure to look at the other medications the patient is taking to make sure that the edema is not a side effect; classic causes of edema include calcium channel blockers, pioglitazone, pregabalin, and NSAIDs.
  - Loops deplete volume in the body, so patients run the risk of not having adequate perfusion through the kidney; elevations in creatinine from baseline can help us monitor for this risk

- Kidney function and electrolytes are going to be the primary labs to monitor
- Urinary output and monitoring of weights can be very important patient factors to monitor and help assess the efficacy of how well the loop diuretic (or any diuretic) is working

Gabapentin (Neurontin)

- Class: Antiepileptic
- Mechanism of Action: Not very clear, but may modulate excitatory neurotransmitters
- Common Uses: Neuropathy, various pain syndromes and other types of nerve pain, seizures
- Memorable Side Effects: Sedation, dizziness, edema
- Clinical Pearls:
  - Generally classified as an anti-seizure medication, but most often used for neuropathy
  - Keep an eye out for patients with kidney disease who may be experiencing side effects as this drug can accumulate in patients with poor renal function
  - Watch out for dizziness and sedation in our elderly patients as this can potentially contribute to falls
  - Weight gain in the form of edema may potentially happen with gabapentin; be on the lookout for patients with a history CHF and edema issues, as well as those who may already be receiving diuretics like furosemide
  - Pregabalin in general has a very similar mechanism of action to gabapentin, so it may also potentially be used (more expensive at this time)

Gemfibrozil (Lopid)

- Class: Antilipemic agent, Fibric acid derivative
- Mechanism of Action: Not well understood, ultimately decreases cholesterol, particularly used for triglycerides
- Common Uses: Elevated Lipids (triglycerides)
- Memorable Side Effects: Dyspepsia (GI), rhabdomyolysis/myopathy possible especially when co-administered with statins
- Clinical Pearls:
  - Interacts with many of the statins, but sometimes used together
  - Important to educate patients, have heightened monitoring for statin adverse effects if using gemfibrozil with a statin
  - Usually twice daily 30 minutes prior to breakfast and dinner
  - GI upset is usually the primary adverse effect

Gentamycin

- Class: Aminoglycoside, Antibiotic
- Mechanism of Action: Blocks bacterial protein synthesis
- Common Uses: Gram negative bacteria; UTI's, sepsis, skin infections
- Memorable Side Effects: CNS changes, diarrhea, kidney impairment, changes in hearing
- Clinical Pearls:
    - Kidney function monitoring is critical – classic nephrotoxic drug
    - Monitoring of drug levels important
    - Usual trough target is less than 2mcg/mL
    - Ototoxicity (ear) is more likely with prolonged use
    - Peak sample usually drawn 30 minutes after infusion complete and trough right before next dose

Glipizide (Amaryl)

- Class: Anti-diabetic agent, Sulfonylurea
- Mechanism of Action: Stimulates pancreatic cells to produce/release insulin
- Common Uses: Diabetes
- Memorable Side Effects: Hypoglycemia, weight gain
- Clinical Pearls:
  - Via its mechanism of action, whenever you increase insulin, hypoglycemia is of highest concern
  - Be attentive to appetite changes or new diabetes medications and monitor for hypoglycemia
  - Often you will see blood sugars bottom out in the early morning when awakening (sleeping is generally the longest period of time when you don't eat)
  - Elderly can be especially at risk for hypoglycemia
  - Weight gain can be problematic in type 2 patients as many likely struggle with metabolic syndrome/weight control already

Glucagon

- Class: Hypoglycemia antidote
- Mechanism of Action: Stimulates adenylate cyclase which results in increased glucose production causing an increase in blood sugar
- Common Uses: Treatment of hypoglycemia
- Memorable Side Effects: Hyperglycemia, change in BP/Pulse, GI
- Clinical Pearls:
  - Be sure patients are educated on how/when to use glucagon
  - If alert without any mental status change, in most cases should be able to oral glucose vs. glucagon
  - Risk of aspiration exists if try to give oral glucose gel (or other source of sugar) to a patient who is in and out of consciousness – so give glucagon in this case
  - Close monitoring of blood glucose is obviously important

Glyburide (Micronase, Diabeta)

- Class: Antidiabetic agent, Sulfonylurea
- Mechanism of Action: Stimulates pancreatic cells to produce/release insulin
- Common Uses: Diabetes
- Memorable Side Effects: Hypoglycemia, weight gain
- Clinical Pearls:
  - Glipizide is usually preferred over glyburide in the elderly if a sulfonylurea is to be used
  - Via its mechanism of action, whenever you increase insulin, hypoglycemia is of highest concern
  - Be attentive to appetite changes or new diabetes medications and monitor for hypoglycemia
  - Often you will see blood sugars bottom out in the early morning when awakening (sleeping is generally the longest period of time when you don't eat)
  - Elderly can be especially at risk for hypoglycemia
  - Weight gain can be problematic in type 2 patients as many likely struggle with metabolic syndrome/weight control already

Guaifenesin (Mucinex)

- Class: Mucous expectorant
- Mechanism of Action: Possibly increases amount of liquid in respiratory tract thereby has an expectorant effect
- Common Uses: Promote loosening of mucus
- Memorable Side Effects: Pretty well tolerated overall
- Clinical Pearls:
  - Some argue that guaifenesin is not an effective expectorant
  - Found in a ton of OTC cough and cold preparations
  - There is an immediate release and extended release product
  - Always important with over the counter medications to educate patients on factors that may help guide them on when to seek medical attention with common cold symptoms (symptoms greater than 7 days, continually worsening symptoms, significant fever, rash, underlying respiratory condition, high risk for complications etc.)

Haloperidol (Haldol)

- Class: Antipsychotic (1st generation)
- Mechanism of Action: Blocks dopamine receptors
- Common Uses: Schizophrenia, Bipolar disorder, (off label - dementia related behaviors like aggression, hallucinations or delusions)
- Memorable Side Effects: Sedation, fall risk, orthostatic BP changes, EPS, metabolic syndrome
- Clinical Pearls:
  - Haloperidol is a first generation antipsychotic and has a very high rate of EPS (movement disorder side effects)
  - Usually higher doses are required for younger patients with schizophrenia and/or bipolar disorder while lower doses can and should be used in the elderly
  - Remember with antipsychotic medications that they block dopamine and can exacerbate conditions where there is a shortage of dopamine like Parkinson's disorder (remember that we use dopamine to treat Parkinson's – i.e. carbidopa/levodopa)
  - Sedation, orthostatic hypotension, movement disorder side effects can all increase the risk of falls especially in our elderly patients
  - NMS (neuroleptic malignant syndrome) is a very rare but very serious complication with antipsychotic medications; a few symptoms of NMS include: fever, hyperreflexia, confusion, delirium, tremor
  - Antipsychotics increase risk of metabolic syndrome (diabetes, elevated lipids, weight gain, etc.) – it is important to periodically monitor for this, especially in younger patients with schizophrenia and/or

bipolar who may be likely to require long term use of higher doses

- o Anticholinergic effects are possible as well with antipsychotics, dry eyes, dry mouth, exacerbation of urinary retention (i.e. BPH), constipation (SLUD – can't salivate, lacrimate, urinate or defecate)
- o Antipsychotics can contribute to QTc prolongation, which can be especially problematic in patients who are already at risk (i.e. on antiarrhythmic medications)

Heparin

- Class: Anticoagulant
- Mechanism of Action: Primarily inactivates thrombin, also may have effects on other clotting factors
- Common Uses: Treatment and prevention of clots, also used in PCI, and to prevent clotting/flush IV lines
- Memorable Side Effects: Bleeding, thrombocytopenia, HIT (rare)
- Clinical Pearls:
  - Bleed risk is top monitoring parameter
  - Risk of thrombocytopenia (heparin induced thrombocytopenia – "HIT") – platelets are very important to monitor
  - Used to flush IV lines (prevent clotting)
  - Many concentrations available (scary for medication error risk)

Hydralazine (Apresoline)

- Class: Vasodilator, Antihypertensive
- Mechanism of Action: Directly dilates arteries and arterioles (decreases BP)
- Common Uses: Hypertension
- Memorable Side Effects: Low BP, CNS changes, exacerbate/contribute to Lupus (rare)
- Clinical Pearls:
  - Fall/orthostatic blood pressure risk
  - Can exacerbate Lupus
  - Dosed multiple times per day so difficult for patients to adhere to medication regimen

Hydrochlorothiazide (Hydrodiuril)

- Class: Antihypertensive, Thiazide Diuretic
- Mechanism of Action: Inhibit sodium/chloride transporter in the distal tubules
- Common Use: hypertension, edema, heart failure
- Memorable Side Effects: (similar to loop diuretics) they are going to increase urine output and decrease amount of volume in the body which can lead to frequent urination, electrolyte depletion, low blood pressure, and increased risk of kidney failure
- Clinical Pearls
  - One of the major differences between loops and thiazides are that thiazides can INCREASE serum calcium while loops will reduce it
  - While loop diuretics can cause hyperuricemia (elevated uric acid possibly contributing to or exacerbating gout), thiazides are classically known to do this – Be on the lookout for hydrochlorothiazide when gout medications are being added or patients are reporting gout flares
  - Hydrochlorothiazide (HCTZ) is used in a ton of medication combinations for hypertension; Examples: Triamterene/HCTZ, Lisinopril/HCTZ etc. This can often confuse patients and they may not realize that they are actually receiving two medications
  - Kidney function and electrolytes are going to be the primary labs to monitor – potassium supplementation is common in patients taking diuretics
  - Watch the timing of diuretics like hydrochlorothiazide – too close to evening can be very problematic as patients will be getting up to go to the bathroom all night

Hydrocodone/acetaminophen (Norco, Lortab)

- Class: Opioid Analgesic – see acetaminophen
- Mechanism of Action: Binds opioid receptors inhibiting CNS pain pathways and causes pain relief; acetaminophen is believed to inhibit prostaglandin production, but does not have anti-inflammatory effects like NSAIDs
- Common Uses: Management of pain disorders, both chronic and acute
- Memorable Side Effects: Constipation, sedation, respiratory depression, CNS effects like confusion, delirium etc., itch, liver toxicity (acetaminophen in large doses >4 grams/day)
- Clinical Pearls:
  - With continuous use of opioid type medication, we have to be assessing constipation and patients will likely require the use of laxatives
  - Be extremely cautious with acetaminophen use and make sure our patient is aware that this product has acetaminophen in it – accidental overdose is a significant problem as acetaminophen is in literally hundreds of over the counter and other prescription products
  - In general, a 3,000 mg (3 gram) max is recommended; 4,000 mg is generally considered safe, and you may see it utilized under certain controlled situations (in adults)
  - Naloxone is reversal agent for opioids
  - I've seen nurses get mixed up on oxycodone and hydrocodone – these medications are not interchangeable!

Hydromorphone (Dilaudid)

- Class: Opioid Analgesic
- Mechanism of Action: Binds opioid receptors inhibiting CNS pain pathways and causes pain relief
- Common Uses: Management of pain disorders, both chronic and acute
- Memorable Side Effects: Constipation, sedation, CNS effects like confusion, delirium etc., respiratory depression
- Clinical Pearls:
  - Hydromorphone is a scheduled 2 controlled substance; risk of addiction, dependence, etc.
  - It is critical to educate/assess patients for constipation if they are taking frequent opioids like hydromorphone
  - Naloxone is reversal agent for opioids
  - Driving/working machinery is certainly risky when using opioids as they can cause significant sedation (usually patients get used to this side effect if they take the medication chronically)

Ibuprofen (Motrin, Advil)

- Class: NSAID, Antipyretic, Analgesic
- Mechanism of Action: Inhibits Cyclooxygenase-1 and 2 (COX-1 and COX-2); results in a reduction in prostaglandins which cause pain, fever, inflammation
- Common Uses: Pain, fever, inflammation
- Memorable Side Effects: GI ulcer, worsening kidney function, edema, hypertension, inhibits platelets (can exacerbate bleed risk)
- Clinical Pearls:
    - NSAIDs are one of the most common causes of GI bleeding; this risk increases in the elderly and those on medications that increase risk of bleeding (anticoagulants and antiplatelet medications)
    - Because of the side effects of GI upset/bleeding, NSAIDs should be taken with food
    - Ibuprofen does have a relatively shorter half-life compared to other NSAIDs and usually needs to be dosed more frequently
    - Due to effects on platelets, NSAIDs are typically held before/after surgery to reduce the risk of bleeding
    - NSAIDs can contribute to edema and exacerbate CHF (congestive heart failure); be on the lookout and have NSAIDs reassessed if you see a patient with a CHF exacerbation or a patient requiring increasing diuretics like furosemide
    - NSAIDs can cause worsening kidney function (creatinine should be monitored); this risk can be greatly increased in patients on ACE Inhibitors or ARBs and/or diuretic type medications
    - Due to above reasons on kidney function, GI bleed risk, and CHF, NSAIDs are not the safest medication

in the elderly (acetaminophen is generally preferred for generalized pain with a few exceptions)

- o Although generally considered more risky in the elderly, a big advantage of NSAIDs over acetaminophen is that they can reduce inflammation
- o Pregnancy category C/D when >30 weeks gestation; NSAIDs are generally avoided in pregnancy and especially after 30 weeks gestation

Infliximab (Remicade)

- Class: Antirheumatic, TNF blocker
- Mechanism of Action: Blocks tumor necrosis factor (TNF) – TNF plays a role in the inflammatory process
- Common Uses: rheumatoid arthritis, psoriasis/psoriatic arthritis, Crohn's, ulcerative colitis
- Memorable Side Effects: Infection risk (suppresses immune system), injection site reaction
- Clinical Pearls:
  - Suppresses immune system (increased risk of serious infections is a boxed warning)
  - Boxed warning for malignancy
  - Increased risk of elevated LFT's especially if used with methotrexate
  - Infusion related side effects

Insulin Aspart (Novolog)

- Class: Rapid acting insulin analog
- Mechanism of Action: Rapid acting insulin causes reduction in blood glucose
- Common Uses: Diabetes
- Memorable Side Effects: Weight gain, hypoglycemia, injection site issues (rotating sites usually alleviates this problem)
- Clinical Pearls:
  - Rapid acting insulin – so you will see this used to quickly bring down blood sugar, compared to the long acting insulins like detemir and glargine
  - Sliding scale insulin is not ideal for diabetes management as you often end up "chasing" blood sugars
  - When giving rapid acting insulin like aspart, remember to be aware of hypoglycemia protocols (juice, glucose gel, saltine crackers etc., or glucagon if patient is incapable of taking oral food/liquid)
  - In many type 2 diabetes patients uncontrolled by oral medications, a combination of long acting once daily with rapid acting insulin with meal(s) is often used
  - With insulin products, some providers will use hold orders on insulin if blood sugars are below a certain value (i.e. 100 mg/dL)
  - Keep an eye out for patients who have a change in appetite as they may require a reduction or increase in insulin based upon their dietary intake

Insulin Detemir (Levemir)

- Class: Long Acting Insulin
- Mechanism of Action: Long acting insulin causes reduction in blood glucose
- Common Uses: Diabetes
- Memorable Side Effects: Weight gain, hypoglycemia, injection site issues (rotating sites usually alleviates this problem)
- Clinical Pearls:
  - Detemir is a long acting, sometimes called "peakless" or "basal" insulin
  - The intent with long acting insulin is to mimic the consistent low level output of insulin by the pancreas
  - Usually dosed once daily, but providers may be more likely to try to do twice daily as the dose increases (more injections for the patient is the downside)
  - Basal insulin in Type 2 diabetes is often (but doesn't have to be) used after patients have tried oral medications without successful decrease in A1C
  - Hypoglycemia is always a concern with any insulin product

Insulin Glargine (Lantus)

- Class: Long Acting Insulin
- Mechanism of Action: Long acting insulin causes reduction in blood glucose
- Common Uses: Diabetes
- Memorable Side Effects: Weight gain, hypoglycemia, injection site issues (rotating sites usually alleviates this problem)
- Clinical Pearls:
  - Glargine is a long acting, sometimes called "peakless" or "basal" insulin
  - The intent with long acting insulin is to mimic the consistent low level output of insulin by the pancreas
  - Usually dosed once daily, but providers may be more likely to try to do twice daily as the dose increases (more injections for the patient is the downside)
  - Basal insulin in Type 2 diabetes is often (but doesn't have to be) used after patients have tried oral medications without successful decrease in A1C
  - Hypoglycemia is always a concern with any insulin product

Insulin Lispro (Humalog)

- Class: Rapid Acting Insulin
- Mechanism of Action: Rapid acting insulin causes reduction in blood glucose
- Common Uses: Diabetes, will see rapid acting used via sliding scale
- Memorable Side Effects: Weight gain, hypoglycemia, injection site issues (rotating sites usually alleviates this problem)
- Clinical Pearls:
  - Rapid acting insulin – so you will see this used to quickly bring down blood sugar, compared to the long acting insulins like detemir and glargine
  - Sliding scale insulin is not ideal for diabetes management as you often end up "chasing" blood sugars
  - When giving rapid acting insulin like aspart, remember to be aware of hypoglycemia protocols (juice, glucose gel, saltine crackers etc., or glucagon if patient is incapable of taking oral food/liquid)
  - In many type 2 diabetes patients uncontrolled by oral medications, a combination of long acting once daily with rapid acting insulin with meal(s) is often used
  - With insulin products, some providers will use hold orders on insulin if blood sugars are below a certain value (i.e. 100 mg/dL)
  - Keep an eye out for patients who have a change in appetite as they may require a reduction or increase in insulin based upon their dietary intake

Irbesartan (Avapro)

- Class: Antihypertensive, ARB
- Mechanism of Action: Blocks the angiotensin 2 receptor – ends up preventing vasoconstriction, aldosterone release etc. (remember aldosterone antagonists can raise potassium just like ARBs and ACE Inhibitors)
- Common Uses: hypertension, heart failure
- Memorable Side Effects: hyperkalemia, exacerbate/worsen kidney function, low blood pressure
- Clinical Pearls:
  - When you think of ARBs and ACE inhibitors, you can lump the side effects together as they are overall the same
  - One major exception to the above rule is the side effect of cough; cough usually doesn't happen with ARBs, and in many patients you will see patients who develop cough on an ACE inhibitor be transitioned to an ARB
  - Kidney function changes and monitoring of potassium is critical when doses are changed or an ARB is initiated
  - This worsening kidney function risk increases in patients who may be taking NSAIDs and/or diuretics
  - As with any medication used to treat hypertension, we need to educate our patients to rise slowly when getting up to minimize risk of orthostatic (sometimes called postural) hypotension

Iron sucrose (Venofer)

- Class: Iron Supplement
- Mechanism of Action: Restoration of iron stores
- Common Uses: Iron deficiency (likely causing anemia)
- Memorable Side Effects: hypotension, GI, anaphylaxis (rare, but serious)
- Clinical Pearls:
  - Risk of anaphylaxis from infusion is a significant risk
  - Ferritin and hemoglobin are important labs to monitor
  - May cause hypotension (BP monitoring important)

Ketorolac (Toradol)

- Class: NSAID, Analgesic
- Mechanism of Action: Inhibits Cyclooxygenase-1 and 2 (COX-1 and COX-2); results in a reduction in prostaglandins which cause pain, fever, inflammation
- Common Uses: Pain, fever, inflammation
- Memorable Side Effects: GI ulcer, worsening kidney function, edema, hypertension, inhibits platelets (can exacerbate bleed risk)
- Clinical Pearls:
  - Injectable available
  - One of the highest risk NSAIDs for GI bleed; this risk increases in the elderly and those on medications that increase risk of bleeding (anticoagulants and antiplatelet medications)
  - Due to effects on platelets, NSAIDs are typically held before/after surgery to reduce the risk of bleeding
  - NSAIDs can contribute to edema and exacerbate CHF (congestive heart failure); be on the lookout and have NSAIDs reassessed if you see a patient with a CHF exacerbation or a patient requiring increasing diuretics like furosemide
  - NSAIDs can cause worsening kidney function (creatinine should be monitored); this risk can be greatly increased in patients on ACE Inhibitors or ARBs and/or diuretic type medications
  - Due to above reasons on kidney function, GI bleed risk, and CHF, NSAIDs are not the safest medication in the elderly (acetaminophen is generally preferred for generalized pain with a few exceptions)
  - Pregnancy category C/D when >30 weeks gestation; NSAIDs are generally avoided in pregnancy and especially after 30 weeks gestation

Lamotrigine (Lamictal)

- Class: Antiepileptic
- Mechanism of Action: Inhibits release of glutamate (excitatory) and inhibits sodium channels
- Common Uses: Seizures, bipolar disorder
- Memorable Side Effects: GI, CNS (drowsiness, dizziness), rash (can be very serious)
- Clinical Pearls:
  o Very slow dosing titration
  o If increase dose too fast, one of the major risks is Steven Johnson's syndrome (very severe, potentially life threatening rash)
  o Does have interactions with other seizure medications (use lower starting dose with valproic acid, higher with enzyme inducers, i.e. phenytoin)
  o Blood levels usually aren't routinely taken

Lansoprazole (Prevacid)

- Class: PPI
- Mechanism of Action: Inhibits proton pumps in the stomach leading to a less acidic environment
- Common Uses: GERD, ulcer, Barrett's esophagus
- Memorable Side Effects: Usually pretty well tolerated; Long term use: Possibility to increase fracture risk, decrease B12 levels, C. diff risk, low magnesium
- Clinical Pearls:
  - PPI's are the most potent acid blocker on the market
  - PPI's are generally dosed 30 minutes or so before meals – this is a recommendation, not an absolute (example if a patient likes to get up and eat right away upon rising, the medication will still likely be beneficial, but may not have a maximal effect)
  - For some patients PPI's may not work very quickly, i.e. it might take a few days for maximal effect
  - For the above reason, as needed (PRN) PPI's can possibly be effective, but are generally not recommended
  - Use short term if possible due to increased risk of osteoporosis, low magnesium, and B12 deficiency if used long term
  - Most common primary outcome of PPI would be to improve symptoms likely heartburn and stomach from GERD, stomach ulcer, or other related condition
  - Barrett's esophagus, high risk GI medications (i.e. NSAIDs, prednisone), or chronic GI bleed may require indefinite therapy
  - If GI bleed is problematic, monitoring hemoglobin and/or hemoccult might be appropriate to assess possible blood loss

Latanoprost (Xalatan)

- Class: Prostaglandin analog
- Mechanism of Action: Prostaglandin F2 alpha analog – decreases intraocular pressure
- Common Uses: Glaucoma
- Memorable Side Effects: Change in eye color, eye irritation
- Clinical Pearls:
  - Generally dosed in the evening for glaucoma
  - Change in eye color may be permanent (change to brown)
  - Many glaucoma patients will be on multiple eye drops – at least 5 minutes is the appropriate amount of time to wait between drops
  - Expires in 42 days once removed from the fridge (REFRIDGERATE until put into use!)

Levofloxacin (Levaquin)

- Class: Quinolone, Antibiotic
- Mechanism of Action: Inhibits bacterial DNA synthesis
- Common Uses: Pneumonia, UTI's, complicated skin infections
- Memorable Side Effects: GI side effects, QTc prolongation (rare)
- Clinical Pearls:
  - Commonly used for both UTI's and Pneumonia
  - Watch out for binding interactions that can decrease absorption (like co-administration with calcium or iron)
  - May increase QTc prolongation risk especially in patients already at risk (on antiarrhythmic medications or other meds that may prolong QTc interval)
  - Spontaneous tendon rupture has been reported (extremely rare)

Levothyroxine (Synthroid)

- Class: Hypothyroid Replacement
- Mechanism of Action: Synthetic T4 hormone, converted to active T3 metabolite
- Common Uses: Replacement hormone for patients with hypothyroidism
- Memorable Side Effects: anxiety, tachycardia, weight loss, decreased bone mineral density, insomnia, GI side effects
- Clinical Pearls:
  - Remember that in patients with hypothyroidism, they will have a lack of energy, fatigue, possible weight gain and many symptoms that might mimic depression
  - If hypothyroidism causes fatigue and lethargy symptoms, remember that giving too much levothyroxine will cause the opposite (i.e. it will ramp up the patient putting them at risk for tachycardia, anxiety etc.)
  - TSH is the major monitoring parameter for levothyroxine dosing – Dosing is counterintuitive! Remember that when TSH is low, it indicates that levothyroxine should be increased; the reason for this is due to a negative feedback loop
  - In practice, I commonly see ½ tabs, and possibly alternating daily doses which can increase risk for errors and confusion
  - Use of calcium supplements is extremely common – giving calcium and levothyroxine together will significantly block the absorption of the levothyroxine, and our patient may require an increase in their levothyroxine dose
  - With administration of levothyroxine, it is generally recommended to give early in the morning prior to

other meds/food etc. HOWEVER if a patient is stabilized (TSH is normal) and doesn't take it this way, it is ok – consistency is the key!

Lisdexamfetamine (Vyvanse)

- Class: CNS Stimulant
- Mechanism of Action: Causes release of dopamine and norepinephrine and may also block reuptake of norepinephrine and dopamine leading to CNS stimulation
- Common Uses: ADHD, depression/fatigue (off label)
- Memorable Side Effects: Anxiety, insomnia, poor appetite, weight loss, hypertension, pulse, emotional lability
- Clinical Pearls:
  - Remembering that this medication ramps you up (stimulant) will help you remember its side effects (anxiety, insomnia, weight loss, poor appetite, increased BP, increased pulse etc.)
  - When used in pediatrics, poor appetite can be a significant problem and should be something that should be assessed
  - BP and Pulse monitoring important
  - Be cautious in patients who may have cardiovascular risk (hypertension etc.)
  - Schedule 2 controlled substance, highly addictive

Lisinopril (Zestril, Prinivil)

- Class: Antihypertensive, ACE Inhibitor
- Mechanism of Action: Lisinopril inhibits angiotensin converting enzyme which prevents the production of angiotensin 2 and leads to lower BP; Angiotensin 2 is a potent vasoconstrictor
- Common Uses: Hypertension, acute MI, heart failure
- Common Side Effects: Cough, kidney impairment, low blood pressure, and hyperkalemia
- Clinical Pearls:
  - ACE Inhibitors are notoriously known for causing a dry chronic cough; if you ever have a patient with a chronic cough, you must assess if they are on an ACE Inhibitor
  - Angiotensin Receptor Blockers (ARBs) are the cousins to the ACE Inhibitors, and are the first line substitute to a patient who has had a cough with an ACE Inhibitor
  - ACE inhibitors can exacerbate kidney impairment as well as contribute to acute renal failure especially in patients who are already on other potential renal toxic medications (i.e. diuretics, NSAIDs etc.) even though in conditions like heart failure, diuretics and ACE Inhibitors are often used together
  - ACE Inhibitors are a classic cause of elevated potassium levels; if your patient has hyperkalemia, you must make sure the ACE Inhibitor has been addressed
  - In some cases, African Americans may not respond to ACE Inhibitors as well as other ethnicities
  - A common mistake I've seen clinicians make is using an ACE Inhibitor with and ARB; this is generally not recommended

- ACE Inhibitors (and ARBs) are frequently used in patients with hypertension and a history of diabetes, stroke, CAD, CKD, and CHF
- Angioedema (swelling of the lips/airway) is classically caused by ACE inhibitors...it is extremely rare, but very serious requiring immediate discontinuation

Lithium (Lithobid)

- Class: Mood Stabilizer, Antimanic Agent
- Mechanism of Action: Not well understood
- Common Uses: Acute and maintenance treatment for bipolar disorder
- Memorable Side Effects: Ataxia, GI, tremor, hypothyroid
- Clinical Pearls:
  - Early toxicity signs – nausea, vomiting, sedation, weakness, difficulty walking or coordinating movements, tremor
  - Risk of seizure/coma with very high levels
  - Kidney function very important to monitor
  - Can impact Thyroid function (monitor TSH)
  - Usually therapeutic level considered 0.5-1.2 mEq/L

Loperamide (Imodium)

- Class: Antidiarrheal
- Mechanism of Action: Acts on opioid receptors on intestines and slows peristalsis (GI movement)
- Common Uses: Diarrhea
- Memorable Side Effects: Constipation, abdominal pain
- Clinical Pearls:
  - Over-the-counter availability
  - Make sure to have patients who use this chronically on their own assessed for other problems (IBS, infection, etc.)
  - Can be used as needed

Lorazepam (Ativan)

- Class: Antianxiety, Benzodiazepine
- Mechanism of Action: enhances activity of GABA (an inhibitor neurotransmitter that causes sedation)
- Common Uses: Anxiety, seizure, insomnia
- Memorable Side Effects: Sedation, confusion, fall risk, dizziness
- Clinical Pearls:
  - The best way I remember benzodiazepines is that they are very close to "alcohol in a pill"
  - Sedation, slurred speech, trouble walking (ataxia) etc. are all common with benzo's/alcohol; they are also commonly used in alcohol withdrawal
  - Be cautious with patients on higher doses of benzodiazepines to make sure they aren't abruptly stopped
  - Educate patients on driving/operating machinery (remember that benzodiazepines are often used for sleep as well as anxiety)
  - Unlike SSRI's for anxiety, a great advantage of benzo's is that they work quickly and can be used as needed
  - Falls in the elderly is a big downside to using these medications
  - Benzo's are a controlled substance, i.e. they can cause addiction, etc.
  - Can be used for acute behavioral issues as well as seizure
  - Flumazenil is antidote in overdose

Losartan (Cozaar)

- Class: Antihypertensive, ARB
- Mechanism of Action: Block the angiotensin 2 receptor – ends up preventing vasoconstriction, aldosterone release, etc. (remember aldosterone antagonists can raise potassium just like ARBs and ACE Inhibitors)
- Common Uses: Hypertension, heart failure
- Memorable Side Effects: Hyperkalemia, exacerbate/worsen kidney function, low blood pressure
- Clinical Pearls:
  - When you think of ARBs and ACE inhibitors, you can lump the side effects together as they are overall the same
  - One major exception to the above rule is the side effect of cough; cough usually doesn't happen with ARBs, and in many patients you will see patients who develop cough on an ACE inhibitor be transitioned to an ARB
  - Kidney function changes and monitoring of potassium is critical when doses are changed or an ARB is initiated
  - This worsening kidney function risk increases in patients who may be taking NSAIDs and/or diuretics
  - As with any medication used to treat hypertension, we need to educate our patients to rise slowly when getting up to minimize risk of orthostatic (sometimes called postural) hypotension

Lovastatin (Mevacor)

- Class: Antilipemic, Statin
- Mechanism of Action: HMG Co-A reductase inhibitor (eventually decreases LDL)
- Common Uses: Reduction of cholesterol (particularly LDL)
- Memorable Side Effects: muscle aches, rhabdomyolysis (rare but serious)
- Clinical Pearls:
  - Statins like lovastatin are one of the mainstays of therapy to reduce cholesterol, and more particularly LDL (bad cholesterol)
  - The most notable side effect with statins that you will likely hear patients complain about is myopathy (muscle aches/pain)
  - Usually muscle aches are all over which can help you differentiate from other pain conditions or pain/soreness from an injury or overuse
  - Contraindicated in pregnancy
  - Patients who do not tolerate lovastatin, may try another statin as long as adverse effects aren't too severe (i.e. rhabdomyolysis); if you notice that the patient had an allergy or intolerance, you need to clarify with the provider
  - CPK will be the primary lab to test for rhabdomyolysis – breakdown of muscle; this elevation in CPK may eventually lead to kidney failure
  - If they are going to, patients usually will present with myopathy when the medication is first started or increased, but be on the lookout for new medications that can interact with statins like CYP3A4 inhibitor drug interactions with classic medications like fluconazole or erythromycin

- For most statins it is "recommended" to give them at night – this is not an absolute, but the drugs ideally work the best when given at night
- Lovastatin is used less frequently because it doesn't reduce LDL as much as newer statins like atorvastatin, simvastatin, and rosuvastatin

Meclizine (Antivert)

- Class: Antiemetic, Antihistamine, Dopamine Blocker
- Mechanism of Action: Blocks dopamine receptors as well as H1 receptors (antiemetic effects, sedation)
- Common Uses: Vertigo (chronic dizziness), nausea/vomiting, motion sickness
- Memorable Side Effects: Sedation, fall risk, orthostatic BP changes, EPS, metabolic syndrome
- Clinical Pearls:
  - Whenever you see an order for meclizine to treat dizziness, be sure to assess other medications (sleepers, psych meds, opioids, antihypertensives, etc.) to make sure they aren't causing/worsening dizziness
  - Can be given as needed
  - Blocks H1 receptors, so sedation will be common
  - Anticholinergic effects, but probably not a major deal if used as needed/infrequently at low doses

Meloxicam (Mobic)

- Class: NSAID, Analgesic
- Mechanism of Action: Inhibits Cyclooxygenase-1 and 2 (COX-1 and COX-2); results in a reduction in prostaglandins which cause pain, fever, inflammation
- Common Uses: Pain, fever, inflammation
- Memorable Side Effects: GI ulcer, worsening kidney function, edema, hypertension, inhibits platelets (can exacerbate bleed risk)
- Clinical Pearls:
  - NSAIDs are one of the most common causes of GI bleeding; this risk increases in the elderly and those on medications that increase risk of bleeding (anticoagulants and antiplatelet medications)
  - Because of the side effects of GI upset/bleeding, NSAIDs should be taken with food
  - Due to effects on platelets, NSAIDs are typically held before/after surgery to reduce the risk of bleeding
  - NSAIDs can contribute to edema and exacerbate CHF (congestive heart failure); be on the lookout and have NSAIDs reassessed if you see a patient with a CHF exacerbation or a patient requiring increasing diuretics like furosemide
  - NSAIDs can cause worsening kidney function (creatinine should be monitored); this risk can be greatly increased in patients on ACE Inhibitors or ARBs and/or diuretic type medications
  - Due to above reasons on kidney function, GI bleed risk, and CHF, NSAIDs are not the safest medication in the elderly (acetaminophen is generally preferred for generalized pain with a few exceptions)
  - Although generally considered more risky in the elderly, a big advantage of NSAIDs over

acetaminophen is that they can reduce inflammation
- Pregnancy category C/D when >30 weeks gestation; NSAIDs are generally avoided in pregnancy and especially after 30 weeks gestation

Memantine (Namenda)

- Class: Anti-dementia, NMDA Antagonist
- Mechanism of Action: Blocks NMDA receptors
- Common Uses: Alzheimer's dementia
- Memorable Side Effects: Changes in behavior, worsening confusion, dizziness
- Clinical Pearls:
  - Remember that medications used for dementia only delay the progression; i.e. they do NOT reverse dementia and at best help slow the process of getting worse
  - Memantine has dose adjustments in kidney disease, so keep an eye out for our patients who may have worsening kidney function (rising creatinine) as the drug may begin to accumulate
  - There is both an extended release and immediate release product available now
  - Memantine has a different mechanism of action from other dementia medications (i.e. donepezil etc.) so it can be used in combination

Metformin (Glucophage)

- Class: Antidiabetic, Biguanide
- Mechanism of Action: Decreases hepatic glucose production (doesn't stimulate production of insulin which is why it is not likely to cause hypoglycemia when used alone)
- Common Uses: Diabetes
- Memorable Side Effects: N/V/D most common, B12 deficiency possible, lactic acidosis (very rare, more common in patients with poor kidney function)
- Clinical Pearls:
  - Metformin is the first line medication for type 2 diabetes
  - Metformin is contraindicated in patients with poor kidney function (serum creatinine >1.4 in females and >1.5 in males); if you know a patient has a history of chronic kidney disease (CKD) make sure use of this medication is reassessed
  - The risk of lactic acidosis increases as this medication is used in the elderly and those with poor kidney function
  - The most common side effect of metformin is GI upset – be on the lookout for patient complaints of this adverse effect and new medication use like PPI's (omeprazole etc.) or other medications that are used to relieve stomach symptoms
  - Administration with a meal is recommended and can really help minimize GI upset
  - Metformin tends to not cause weight gain compared to other diabetes medications which is nice considering that many of our type 2 diabetes patients are overweight

Methadone (Methadose, Dolophine)

- Class: Opioid, Analgesic
- Mechanism of Action: Binds opioid receptors inhibiting CNS pain pathways and causes pain relief
- Common Uses: Management of pain disorders, both chronic and acute, opioid detoxification
- Memorable Side Effects: Constipation, sedation, CNS effects like confusion, delirium etc., respiratory depression
- Clinical Pearls:
  - Methadone is a scheduled 2 controlled substance; risk of addiction, dependence, etc.
  - Used in methadone maintenance programs for treatment of opioid addiction
  - It is critical to educate/assess patients for constipation if they are taking frequent opioids like methadone
  - Naloxone is reversal agent for opioids
  - Driving/working machinery is certainly risky when using opioids as they can cause significant sedation (usually patients get used to this side effect if they take the medication chronically)
  - QTc Prolongation is a risk especially with other medications that can contribute to QTc prolongation (amiodarone, etc.)

Methotrexate (Rheumatrex)

- Class: DMARD (Disease modifying antirheumatic drug), Antineoplastic Agent
- Mechanism of Action: Binds dihydrofolate reductase – in treatment of Rheumatoid arthritis, likely benefit from suppressing the immune system
- Common Uses: Rheumatoid arthritis, psoriasis, certain cancers (much higher doses used in cancer treatment)
- Memorable Side Effects: Low WBC or platelet count, increased liver enzymes
- Clinical Pearls:
    - DMARDs are first line for rheumatoid arthritis
    - Usually dosed once weekly
    - Need to supplement folic acid when using chronically
    - Likely will not be beneficial in acute flare of inflammation (NSAIDs or prednisone typically used for acute RA flare)
    - Suppresses immune system so WBC and infection monitoring is important
    - LFT's should also be monitored

Methylphenidate (Ritalin, Concerta)

- Class: CNS Stimulant
- Mechanism of Action: Blocks reuptake of norepinephrine and dopamine leading to CNS stimulation
- Common Uses: ADHD, depression/fatigue (off label)
- Memorable Side Effects: Anxiety, insomnia, poor appetite, weight loss, hypertension, elevated pulse, emotional lability
- Clinical Pearls:
  - Remembering that this medication ramps you up (stimulant) will help you remember its side effects (anxiety, insomnia, weight loss, poor appetite, increased BP, increased pulse etc.)
  - When used in pediatrics, poor appetite can be a significant problem and should be something that is assessed
  - BP and Pulse monitoring important
  - Be cautious in patients who may have cardiovascular risk (hypertension etc.)
  - Schedule 2 controlled substance, highly addictive

Methylprednisolone (Medrol)

- Class: Corticosteroid
- Mechanism of Action: Suppresses leukocytes and ultimately reduces inflammation, suppresses adrenal function and the immune system
- Common Uses: Acute inflammatory states (dermatitis, arthritis flare, Crohn's, pneumonia, asthma exacerbation etc.)
- Memorable Side Effects: GI side effects, insomnia, hyperglycemia, long term use; suppress immune system, increase osteoporosis risk as well as cause adrenal insufficiency
- Clinical Pearls:
  - Most common use I've seen is a Medrol Dose Pak which is used for relief of short term inflammation related issues
  - Be sure to take steroids with food as they can be pretty hard on the GI tract
  - In patients with diabetes, educate them that a fluctuation in blood sugars may occur when starting, changing doses, or discontinuing this medication due to the adverse effect of hyperglycemia
  - Long term corticosteroid use can lead to increased risk Cushing's (moon face), diabetes, and osteoporosis; make sure long term use is assessed frequently to minimize length and dose of steroids
  - In patients on long term use, they should be assessed if vitamin D and/or calcium and bisphosphonates should be added to reduce osteoporosis risk
  - Insomnia is common in the short term, but may resolve as short term use goes to longer term use

- Short "bursts" (3 days to a week or 2) are often used to relieve acute inflammatory states causing patient distress (asthma, rheumatoid arthritis, etc.)
- Corticosteroids (especially long term and higher doses) can suppress the immune system

Metoclopramide (Reglan)

- Class: Antiemetic, Prokinetic
- Mechanism of Action: Blocks dopamine and serotonin receptors (in CRZ – chemoreceptor zone, lends to relief of nausea/vomiting)
- Common Uses: Gastroparesis (often caused by diabetes), nausea/vomiting
- Memorable Side Effects: Extrapyramidal symptoms
- Clinical Pearls:
  - Has dopamine blocking activity like antipsychotics, so can cause movement disorders like EPS and tardive dyskinesia
  - As above with dopamine blocking activity, not a great choice in a patient with a preexisting movement disorder (i.e. Parkinson's)
  - Most commonly used for gastroparesis (slow moving GI tract) – be on the lookout for anticholinergic medications which can worsen gastroparesis
  - Usually dosed multiple times per day (3-4)

Metoprolol succinate (Toprol XL)

- Class: Antihypertensive, Beta-blocker
- Mechanism of Action: Blocks beta receptors leading to lower pulse/BP
- Common Uses: Hypertension, Atrial fibrillation
- Memorable Side Effects: Low pulse, low BP, fatigue
- Clinical Pearls:
  - Common error in practice I've seen is confusion with metoprolol succinate (Toprol XL) vs metoprolol tartrate (Lopressor); usually dosed once daily, (not always) Succinate is the "sustained" release formulation while tartrate is the immediate release formulation and usually dosed twice daily.
  - Trick to remembering beta receptors: You have 1 heart and 2 lungs (beta-1 is primarily on the heart and beta-2 primarily in the lungs). You will see beta receptors again with respiratory medications. If beta-1 is stimulated, heart rate increases. If beta-1 is blocked, heart rate decreases.
  - The selectivity of these drugs is really important; metoprolol is beta-1 selective, so in a patient with asthma, we would likely not see much of a problem however this selectivity may start to disappear as you push the doses higher
  - Pulse and blood pressure are going to be the two most important monitoring parameters you will want to follow
  - Often in practice, providers will place a hold order on beta-blockers if the pulse is too low. This is obviously done to reduce the risk of significant bradycardia; clinically it may depend upon the situation, but in an ambulatory setting, you may see the order set to hold the beta blocker when pulse is less than 55 or 60.

Metronidazole (Flagyl)

- Class: Antibiotic
- Mechanism of Action: Interferes with bacterial DNA and can inhibit protein synthesis
- Common Uses: C. diff, H. pylori, anaerobic infections (gut infections), bacterial vaginosis
- Memorable Side Effects: GI side effects, metallic taste
- Clinical Pearls:
  - Usual first line treatment for C. diff (oral vancomycin is another common option)
  - Can be utilized for anaerobic bacteria
  - Commonly used in combo in treatment of Helicobacter pylori (H. pylori is a common cause of GI ulcers)
  - NO ALCOHOL with this medication – causes disulfiram reaction
  - IV and PO available

Midazolam (Versed)

- Class: Benzodiazepine, sedative
- Mechanism of Action: enhances activity of GABA (an inhibitor neurotransmitter that causes sedation)
- Common Uses: Sedation/amnesia for procedures in a hospitalized patient, Seizures
- Memorable Side Effects: Sedation, confusion, fall risk, dizziness, amnesia, respiratory depression
- Clinical Pearls:
    - Injectable/IV
    - Primary use is to cause sedation and amnesia in the hospital setting for various procedures/surgery
    - Monitoring of respirations will be important as cases of respiratory arrest have been reported
    - Can be used for surgery as well as seizure
    - Flumazenil is antidote in overdose

Milk of Magnesia

- Class: Laxative
- Mechanism of Action: Increases fluid in the GI tract which stimulates peristaltic activity
- Common Uses: Constipation
- Memorable Side Effects: Elevated magnesium, loose stools
- Clinical Pearls:
  - Watch out for accumulation in CKD (magnesium) – usually not an issue if used infrequently
  - Can be used as needed

Mirtazapine (Remeron)

- Class: Antidepressant
- Mechanism of Action: Blocks alpha 2 which increases norepinephrine and serotonin; also antagonist at certain serotonin receptors and H1 receptors
- Common Uses: Depression, insomnia, anorexia
- Memorable Side Effects: sedation, weight gain (can be good or bad), CNS effects
- Clinical Pearls:
  - Can be used to help with sleep (tends to be more sedating at lower doses) – H1 blocking effects
  - Weight gain can be a problem in younger patients, but can be a positive in frail elderly
  - Not likely to be beneficial as needed (takes weeks to work for depression or anxiety)
  - Sedative properties may work in the short term (as needed)

Mometasone (Nasonex)

- Class: Nasal Corticosteroid
- Mechanism of Action: Nasal steroid that helps reduce inflammation
- Common Uses: Allergies
- Memorable Side Effects: Pretty well tolerated, likely nasal irritation, possible nose bleeds if any
- Clinical Pearls:
  - Gently shake the product for nasal inhalation and you may need to prime the nasal delivery device if it is the first time using it
  - Educate patients that it may not work right away, it may take a few hours or up to a day or two to start working (because of this, it may not be the best to use this as needed, but I've certainly seen it prescribed this way before)
  - It may only be necessary to use this medication seasonally based upon timing and duration of allergy symptoms
  - Be sure to educate patients to clean the tip of the nasal delivery device as it can get pretty nasty!

Montelukast (Singulair)

- Class: Leukotriene receptor blocker
- Mechanism of Action: Blocks leukotriene receptors which can help reduce inflammation
- Common Uses: asthma, allergic rhinitis
- Memorable Side Effects: Pretty well tolerated; Rare – psychiatric or unusual behavior changes
- Clinical Pearls:
  - Usually dosed in the evening, however in patients with ONLY allergies, they may give it at the time of day that works the best
  - Overall, usually pretty well tolerated
  - This medication is meant to control asthma, NOT provide acute relief with an exacerbation (albuterol is used for an asthma attack)
  - Rare post-marketing case reports of neuropsychiatric problems (abnormal behavior, aggression, depression etc.)

Morphine (MS Contin, Oramorph)

- Class: Opioid, Analgesic
- Mechanism of Action: Binds opioid receptors inhibiting CNS pain pathways and causes pain relief
- Common Uses: Management of pain disorders, both chronic and acute
- Memorable Side Effects: Constipation, sedation, CNS effects like confusion, delirium etc., respiratory depression
- Clinical Pearls:
  - Morphine is a scheduled 2 controlled substance; risk of addiction, dependence etc.
  - Very frequently used short term for pain and post-op procedures
  - It is critical to educate/assess patients for constipation if they are taking frequent opioids like morphine
  - Driving/working machinery is certainly risky when using opioids as they can cause significant sedation (usually patients get used to this side effect if they take the medication chronically)
  - MS Contin is the brand name of the extended release morphine
  - Naloxone is reversal agent for opioids
  - You should not see MS Contin used on an as needed basis as it is intended to have a slower/steady absorption over a longer period of time
  - Very high risk for significant error as different liquid concentrations are available – be careful!!

Moxifloxacin (Avelox)

- Class: Quinolone, Antibiotic
- Mechanism of Action: Inhibits bacterial DNA synthesis
- Common Uses: Pneumonia, complicated skin infections
- Memorable Side Effects: GI side effects, QTc prolongation (rare)
- Clinical Pearls:
  - Typically used only for pneumonia (different from ciprofloxacin and levofloxacin)
  - Watch out for binding interactions that can decrease absorption (like co-administration with calcium or iron)
  - May increase QTc prolongation risk especially in patients already at risk (on antiarrhythmic medications or other meds that may prolong QTc interval)
  - Spontaneous tendon rupture has been reported (extremely rare)

Nabumetone (Relafen)

- Class: NSAID, Analgesic
- Mechanism of Action: Inhibits Cyclooxygenase-1 and 2 (COX-1 and COX-2); results in a reduction in prostaglandins which cause pain, fever, inflammation
- Common Uses: Pain, fever, inflammation
- Memorable Side Effects: GI ulcer, worsening kidney function, edema, hypertension, inhibits platelets (can exacerbate bleed risk)
- Clinical Pearls:
  - NSAIDs are one of the most common causes of GI bleeding; this risk increases in the elderly and those on medications that increase risk of bleeding (anticoagulants and antiplatelet medications)
  - Because of the side effects of GI upset/bleeding, NSAIDs should be taken with food
  - Due to effects on platelets, NSAIDs are typically held before/after surgery to reduce the risk of bleeding
  - NSAIDs can contribute to edema and exacerbate CHF (congestive heart failure); be on the lookout and have NSAIDs reassessed if you see a patient with a CHF exacerbation or a patient requiring increasing diuretics like furosemide
  - NSAIDs can cause worsening kidney function (creatinine should be monitored); this risk can be greatly increased in patients on ACE Inhibitors or ARBs and/or diuretic type medications
  - Due to above reasons on kidney function, GI bleed risk, and CHF, NSAIDs are not the safest medication in the elderly (acetaminophen is generally preferred for generalized pain with a few exceptions)
  - Although generally considered more risky in the elderly, a big advantage of NSAIDs over

acetaminophen is that they can reduce inflammation

- o Pregnancy category C/D when >30 weeks gestation; NSAIDs are generally avoided in pregnancy and especially after 30 weeks gestation

Naproxen (Naprosyn, Aleve)

- Class: NSAID, Analgesic
- Mechanism of Action: Inhibits Cyclooxygenase-1 and 2 (COX-1 and COX-2); results in a reduction in prostaglandins which cause pain, fever, inflammation
- Common Uses: Pain, fever, inflammation
- Memorable Side Effects: GI ulcer, worsening kidney function, edema, hypertension, inhibits platelets (can exacerbate bleed risk)
- Clinical Pearls:
  - NSAIDs are one of the most common causes of GI bleeding; this risk increases in the elderly and those on medications that increase risk of bleeding (anticoagulants and antiplatelet medications)
  - Because of the side effects of GI upset/bleeding, NSAIDs should be taken with food
  - Due to effects on platelets, NSAIDs are typically held before/after surgery to reduce the risk of bleeding
  - NSAIDs can contribute to edema and exacerbate CHF (congestive heart failure); be on the lookout and have NSAIDs reassessed if you see a patient with a CHF exacerbation or a patient requiring increasing diuretics like furosemide
  - NSAIDs can cause worsening kidney function (creatinine should be monitored); this risk can be greatly increased in patients on ACE Inhibitors or ARBs and/or diuretic type medications
  - Due to above reasons on kidney function, GI bleed risk, and CHF, NSAIDs are not the safest medication in the elderly (acetaminophen is generally preferred for generalized pain with a few exceptions)
  - Although generally considered more risky in the elderly, a big advantage of NSAIDs over

acetaminophen is that they can reduce inflammation

- ○ Pregnancy category C/D when >30 weeks gestation; NSAIDs are generally avoided in pregnancy and especially after 30 weeks gestation

Nebivolol (Bystolic)

- Class: Antihypertensive, Beta-blocker
- Mechanism of Action: Blocks beta receptors leading to lower pulse/BP
- Common Uses: Hypertension, Atrial fibrillation
- Memorable Side Effects: Low pulse, low BP, fatigue
- Clinical Pearls:
  - Trick to remembering beta receptors: You have 1 heart and 2 lungs (beta-1 is primarily on the heart and beta-2 primarily in the lungs). If beta-1 is stimulated, heart rate increases; if beta-1 is blocked, heart rate decreases
  - Usually only dosed once daily which is a nice advantage over some other beta-blockers
  - Often in practice, providers will place a hold order on beta-blockers if the pulse is too low; this is done to reduce the risk of significant bradycardia
  - Clinically it may depend upon the situation, but in an ambulatory setting, you may see the order set to hold the beta blocker when pulse is less than 55 or 60

Niacin (Niaspan)

- Class: Antilipemic
- Mechanism of Action: Converted to nicotinamide which can affect lipid metabolism
- Common Uses: Hyperlipidemia
- Memorable Side Effects: Flushing, GI, increase uric acid
- Clinical Pearls:
  - Flushing from niacin can be treated with aspirin
  - Slow release formulation may help minimize flushing as well
  - Can possibly exacerbate gout (increase uric acid)
  - Possibly can increase blood sugars, but usually not clinically significant – if a patient had persistent high blood sugars, might be a good idea to avoid niacin
  - Rare possibility of liver issues

Nifedipine (Procardia)

- Class: Antihypertensive, Calcium Channel Blocker
- Mechanism of Action: blocks calcium ions from entering voltage smooth muscle, resulting in relaxation (vasodilation) – dihydropyridine calcium channel blocker
- Common Uses: hypertension
- Memorable Side Effects: low blood pressure, edema, constipation
- Clinical Pearls:
  - Very important distinction: You will not see nifedipine used in atrial fibrillation, because its activity is primarily on the vessels; this differs from non-dihydropyridine calcium channel blockers like verapamil and diltiazem that act on the heart AND blood vessels; This also means that pulse monitoring will not be necessary with nifedipine
  - The higher you push the dose on these medications, the more likely you will see the side effect of edema
  - Keep an eye out for new requirement of diuretic Rx's to treat the edema caused by the calcium channel blockers
  - Educate our patients to get up slowly to minimize risk of orthostatic hypotension
  - Nifedipine has an extended release formulation available

Nitrofurantoin (Macrobid)

- Class: Antibiotic
- Mechanism of Action: Inhibits bacterial protein synthesis, metabolism, DNA, RNA, and cell wall synthesis
- Common Uses: Urinary tract infection
- Memorable Side Effects: GI, CNS (more likely in elderly), neuropathy(rare), pulmonary distress (rare)
- Clinical Pearls:
  - Have use reassessed if patient has kidney disease (contraindicated)
  - May discolor urine – be sure to educate patients on this (brown/orange color)
  - Rare adverse effect of respiratory issues
  - Generally not first line in the elderly for UTI's
  - Category B (so potential option in pregnancy)

Nitroglycerine (Nitrostat)

- Class: Antihypertensive, Antianginal, Nitrate
- Mechanism of Action: Metabolized into nitric oxide which leads to smooth muscle relaxation (vasodilation)
- Common Uses: angina (chest pain)
- Memorable Side Effects: Low BP, headache
- Clinical Pearls:
  - Sublingual used most commonly for acute relief of chest pain (angina)
  - Make sure patients are well educated on chest pain that doesn't resolve with use (emergency)
  - Recommended to only use 3 tablets every 5 minutes (max of 3 tabs)
  - Also long acting products available dosed daily (isosorbide mononitrate) or multiple times daily (isosorbide dinitrate)
  - Patch formulation available as well for those that have trouble swallowing or tolerating the oral formulation

Nitroprusside (Nitropress)

- Class: Antihypertensive, Vasodilator
- Mechanism of Action: Direct vasodilation on vessel smooth muscle
- Common Uses: Hypertensive crisis, heart failure
- Memorable Side Effects: Low blood pressure, changes in heart rate, dizziness, metabolic acidosis
- Clinical Pearls:
  - Drops blood pressure – risk of too much drug is low blood pressure
  - Injection type reaction can happen - pain, redness, rash, warmth
  - Cyanide toxicity is a black box warning if used at too high of a dose or for too long

Norepinephrine (Levophed)

- Class: Alpha and Beta agonist
- Mechanism of Action: Stimulates alpha and beta receptors
- Common Uses: Treatment of shock (severe hypotension)
- Memorable Side Effects: hypertension, arrhythmias, anxiety
- Clinical Pearls:
  - Clamps down on vessels causing an increase in BP
  - Chest pain possible due to reduced blood flow through the heart
  - Boxed warning for extravasation

Nortriptyline (Pamelor)

- Class: TCA, Antidepressant
- Mechanism of Action: Tri-cyclic antidepressant (highly anticholinergic) – inhibits reuptake of serotonin and possibly norepinephrine
- Common Uses: Depression, neuropathy, pain syndromes, anxiety, PTSD
- Memorable Side Effects: Anticholinergic + confusion, fall risk in elderly
- Clinical Pearls:
  - Old TCA generally not recommended in the elderly due to anticholinergic effects (remember anti – SLUDs; can't salivate, lacrimate, urinate, or defecate)
  - In addition, cognitive impairment is not a good thing in the elderly due to possibility of preexisting dementia
  - TCA's may have some benefit in neuropathy, generally much cheaper than SNRI's which are can be beneficial in neuropathy
  - Not a good first line choice for sleep or depression (other agents exist that are much safer)
  - Considered a more tolerable choice than amitriptyline in the elderly
  - Look out for TCA's causing the prescribing cascade! Artificial tears for dry eyes, constipation medications, BPH medications like tamsulosin, dementia medications, or artificial saliva

Olanzapine (Zyprexa)

- Class: Antipsychotic
- Mechanism of Action: Blocks dopamine receptors
- Common Uses: Schizophrenia, Bipolar disorder, dementia related behaviors like aggression, hallucinations, delusions (off-label)
- Memorable Side Effects: Sedation, fall risk, orthostatic BP changes, EPS, metabolic syndrome
- Clinical Pearls:
  - Usually higher doses are required for younger patients with schizophrenia and/or bipolar disorder while lower doses can and should be used in the elderly
  - Remember with antipsychotic medications that they block dopamine and can exacerbate conditions where there is a shortage of dopamine like Parkinson's disorder (remember that we use dopamine to treat Parkinson's – i.e. carbidopa/levodopa or pramipexole)
  - Sedation, orthostatic hypotension, movement disorder side effects can all increase the risk of falls especially in our elderly patients
  - NMS (neuroleptic malignant syndrome) is a very rare but very serious complication with antipsychotic medications; a few symptoms of NMS include: fever, hyperreflexia, confusion, delirium, tremor
  - Antipsychotics increase risk of metabolic syndrome (diabetes, elevated lipids, weight gain etc.) – it is important to periodically monitor for this, especially in younger patients with schizophrenia and/or bipolar who may be likely to require long term use of higher doses; Olanzapine is one of the worst antipsychotics as far as this side effect goes

- o Anticholinergic effects are possible as well with antipsychotics, dry eyes, dry mouth, exacerbation of urinary retention (i.e. BPH), constipation (SLUD – can't salivate, lacrimate, urinate or defecate)
- o Antipsychotics can contribute to QTc prolongation, which can be especially problematic in patients who are already at risk (i.e. on antiarrhythmic medications)

Olmesartan (Benicar)

- Class: Antihypertensive, ARB
- Mechanism of Action: Block the angiotensin 2 receptor – ends up preventing vasoconstriction, aldosterone release etc. (remember aldosterone antagonists can raise potassium just like ARBs and ACE Inhibitors)
- Common Uses: hypertension, heart failure
- Memorable Side Effects: hyperkalemia, exacerbate/worsen kidney function, low blood pressure
- Clinical Pearls:
  - When you think of ARBs and ACE inhibitors, you can lump the side effects together as they are overall the same; one major exception to this rule is the side effect of cough
  - Kidney function changes and monitoring of potassium is critical when doses are changed or an ARB is initiated
  - Orthostatic BP and/or dizziness upon rising is important to ask patients about
  - Risk of kidney injury increases when patients are also on an NSAID and/or Diuretic(s)
  - You shouldn't ever see an ACE Inhibitor (i.e. Lisinopril) and an ARB used together
  - Hyperkalemia risk will increase when using potassium supplements, ACE inhibitors, or potassium sparing diuretics with ARBs

Olopatadine (Patanol)

- Class: Ophthalmic antihistamine
- Mechanism of Action: Histamine receptor blocker (eye drops)
- Common Uses: Allergies where eyes are affected
- Memorable Side Effects: eye irritation
- Clinical Pearls:
  - Blocks histamine receptors, so dry eye is a possibility
  - At least 5 minutes between other eye drops is ideal
  - May only need to use this medication seasonally depending upon allergies

Omeprazole (Prilosec)

- Class: PPI
- Mechanism of Action: Inhibits proton pumps in the stomach leading to a less acidic environment
- Common Uses: GERD, ulcer, Barrett's esophagus
- Memorable Side Effects: Usually pretty well tolerated; Long term use: Possibility to increase fracture risk, decrease B12 levels, C. diff risk, low magnesium
- Clinical Pearls:
  - PPI's are the most potent acid blocker on the market
  - PPI's are generally dosed 30 minutes or so before meals – this is a recommendation, not an absolute (example if a patient likes to get up and eat right away upon rising, the medication will still likely be beneficial, but may not have a maximal effect)
  - For some patients PPI's may not work very quickly, i.e. it might take a few days for maximal effect (this is a disadvantage compared to other acid blocking agents)
  - For the above reason, as needed (PRN) PPI's can possibly be effective, but are generally not recommended
  - Use short term if possible due to increased risk of osteoporosis, low magnesium, and B12 deficiency if used long term
  - Most common primary outcome of PPI would be to improve symptoms likely heartburn and stomach from GERD, stomach ulcer, or other related condition
  - Barrett's esophagus, high risk GI medications (i.e. NSAIDs, prednisone), or chronic GI bleed are a few examples where a patient may require indefinite therapy

- If GI bleed is problematic, monitoring hemoglobin and/or hemoccult might be appropriate to assess possible blood loss

Ondansetron (Zofran)

- Class: Antiemetic, Serotonin receptor antagonist
- Mechanism of Action: Blocks serotonin at 5HT3 receptors – acts centrally in the chemoreceptor trigger zone
- Common Uses: Nausea/vomiting
- Memorable Side Effects: Constipation, sedation, QTc prolongation is a risk (pretty rare unless on other drugs that can contribute to QTc prolongation)
- Clinical Pearls:
  - Frequently used in patients undergoing chemotherapy (nausea/vomiting common with chemo)
  - Can be used as needed or scheduled
  - Can cause QTc prolongation especially when used in combo with other QTc prolonging agents
  - Has serotonin activity, be on the lookout for other serotonergic medications (like SSRI's, tramadol etc.)

Oseltamivir (Tamiflu)

- Class: Antiviral, Neuraminidase Inhibitor
- Mechanism of Action: Inhibits viral neuraminidase, preventing influenza virus from replicating
- Common Uses: Influenza treatment and prophylaxis
- Memorable Side Effects: GI, psych events like delirium (rare, more likely in pediatrics)
- Clinical Pearls:
  - Drug of choice for influenza prophylaxis or treatment
  - Prophylaxis is especially common for patients at high risk who've been exposed to infected individuals (immunosuppressed, elderly, healthcare institution – i.e. nursing home)
  - Dose adjustments in patients with poor kidney function
  - GI upset is going to be the most common side effect
  - With or without food is ok, but likely better tolerated by the stomach with food
  - Encourage influenza vaccination!

Oxybutynin (Ditropan)

- Class: Bladder Anticholinergic
- Mechanism of Action: Blocks muscarinic receptors (anticholinergic) in the bladder which increases urine volume in the bladder and potentially decreases frequency/urge
- Common Uses: Overactive bladder, bladder spasms
- Memorable Side Effects: Anticholinergic effects possible (i.e. can't spit, see, pee or poop - dry mouth, dry eyes, urinary retention, constipation)
- Clinical Pearls:
  - Anticholinergic effects (oxybutynin is highly anticholinergic)
  - Tolterodine is less likely to cause anticholinergic effects than older bladder agents like oxybutynin (more selective for the bladder)
  - Be sure to assess if the medication is working for incontinence/frequency – many patients don't benefit
  - Keep an eye out for patients on diuretics and if urinary frequency is the major issue, make sure that they are minimized if possible (not always possible to reduce diuretics with CHF history, etc.)
  - Frequency can be especially problematic in patients who have an active social life as well as night when trying to sleep
  - Oxybutynin has a patch formulation available (usually twice weekly)

Oxycodone (Oxycontin, Oxyfast, Oxy IR)

- Class: Opioid, Analgesic
- Mechanism of Action: Binds opioid receptors inhibiting CNS pain pathways and causes pain relief
- Common Uses: Management of pain disorders, both chronic and acute
- Memorable Side Effects: Constipation, sedation, respiratory depression, CNS effects like confusion, delirium etc.
- Clinical Pearls:
  o Oxycodone is a scheduled 2 controlled substance; risk of addiction, dependence etc.
  o Very frequently used short term for pain and post-op procedures
  o It is critical to educate/assess patients for constipation if they are taking frequent opioids like oxycodone
  o Naloxone is reversal agent for opioids
  o Driving/working machinery is certainly risky when using opioids as they can cause significant sedation (usually patients get used to this side effect if they take the medication chronically)
  o Hydrocodone and oxycodone are NOT interchangeable – I have seen nurses make this mistake on a number of different occasions as they do look alike and sound alike as well as have similar doses
  o Oxycontin is the brand name of the extended release oxycodone
  o You should not see Oxycontin (oxycodone ER) used on an as needed basis as it is intended to have a slower/steady absorption over a longer period of time

- Oxycodone ER is usually dosed twice daily, occasionally patients may need three times daily if pain is increasing as drug is wearing off
- If the immediate release formulation is used in an institutional setting, be sure that parameters are set up (usually based upon pain scale) – i.e. if pain is 1-5 give 1 tablet and if pain is 6-10 give 2 tablets

Oxycodone/APAP (Percocet)

- Class: Opioid, Analgesic – see acetaminophen
- Mechanism of Action: Binds opioid receptors inhibiting CNS pain pathways and causes pain relief; acetaminophen is believed to inhibit prostaglandin production, but does not have anti-inflammatory effects like NSAIDs
- Common Uses: Management of pain disorders, both chronic and acute
- Memorable Side Effects: Constipation, sedation, respiratory depression, CNS effects like confusion, delirium etc., liver toxicity (acetaminophen in large doses >4 grams/day)
- Clinical Pearls:
  - Risk of acetaminophen overdose is certainly a possibility – need to educate patients that this contains acetaminophen as well as many common OTC's, cough and cold medicines, etc.
  - Oxycodone is a scheduled 2 controlled substance; risk of addiction, dependence, etc.
  - Very frequently used short term for pain and post-op procedures
  - It is critical to educate/assess patients for constipation if they are taking frequent opioids like oxycodone
  - Naloxone is reversal agent for opioids
  - Driving/working machinery is certainly risky when using opioids as they can cause significant sedation (usually patients get used to this side effect if they take the medication chronically)
  - Hydrocodone and oxycodone are NOT interchangeable – I have seen nurses make this mistake on a number of different occasions as they

do look alike and sound alike as well as have similar doses

- o Oxycodone/acetaminophen is meant for acute pain relief and certainly can and is used on a prn (as needed) basis
- o In an institutional setting, be sure that parameters are set up (usually based upon pain scale) – i.e. if pain is 1-5 give 1 tablet and if pain is 6-10 give 2 tablets

Pantoprazole (Protonix)

- Class: PPI
- Mechanism of Action: Inhibits proton pumps in the stomach leading to a less acidic environment
- Common Uses: GERD, ulcer, Barrett's esophagus
- Memorable Side Effects: Usually pretty well tolerated; Long term use: Possibility to increase fracture risk, decrease B12 levels, C. diff risk, low magnesium
- Clinical Pearls:
  - PPI's are the most potent acid blocker on the market
  - PPI's are generally dosed 30 minutes or so before meals – this is a recommendation, not an absolute (example if a patient likes to get up and eat right away upon rising, the medication will still likely be beneficial, but may not have a maximal effect)
  - For some patients PPI's may not work very quickly, i.e. it might take a few days for maximal effect
  - For the above reason, as needed (PRN) PPI's can possibly be effective, but are generally not used
  - Use short term if possible due to increased risk of osteoporosis, low magnesium, and B12 deficiency if used long term
  - Barrett's esophagus, high risk GI medications (i.e. NSAIDs, prednisone), or chronic GI bleed may require indefinite therapy
  - If GI bleed is problematic, monitoring hemoglobin and/or hemoccult might be appropriate to assess possible blood loss

Paroxetine (Paxil)

- Class: Antidepressant, SSRI
- Mechanism of Action: SSRI – selective serotonin reuptake inhibitor; increases serotonin in the brain
- Common Uses: Depression, anxiety, PTSD
- Memorable Side Effects: GI side effects (N/V/D), can really cause sedation or activation depending upon the patient, changes in mental status, hyponatremia (rare)
- Clinical Pearls:
  - SSRI's are generally considered the first line medication to treat depression, they are generally well tolerated, and less risky than other antidepressants in the situation of attempted suicide by overdosing on pills
  - Constipation may be a little more common with paroxetine versus other SSRI's
  - There may be an increased risk of suicidal thinking when first starting these medications (there is a BOXED warning for this risk)
  - Paroxetine tends to be a little more sedating than other SSRI's like sertraline or fluoxetine
  - Although not terribly common, hyponatremia (low sodium) is a possible unique side effect with SSRI's and much more likely in patients already prone to hyponatremia – classic example would be patients who are taking diuretics, which can also lower sodium
  - Remember that these drugs are not an immediate fix! In most cases, SSRI's take weeks sometimes months before a patient will start improving; however side effects will be apparent from the start of the medication, making it difficult to coach our patients to continue the medication in the first few weeks after starting it

- SSRI's are used in pregnancy, but the risk versus the benefits need to be assessed on a case by case basis (paroxetine is actually category D)
- SSRI's can decrease libido

Pegfilgrastim (Neulasta)

- Class: Colony Stimulating Factor (CSF)
- Mechanism of Action: Stimulates production of WBC's
- Common Uses: Prevention of neutropenia in chemo patients
- Memorable Side Effects: Ostealgia (bone pain), anaphylaxis (rare)
- Clinical Pearls:
  - Helps patients continue on chemotherapy by increasing white blood cells and decreasing risk of infection
  - Bone pain is common and you will often see use of NSAIDs and/or acetaminophen used to help treat this (remember that it stimulates bone marrow which resides inside the bones – source of pain)
  - CBC (white blood cell count is incredibly important to monitor for positive response)
  - Fever and signs of infection are also incredibly important to watch for in a patient on pegfilgrastim
  - Long acting version of filgrastim (dosed less frequently)

Penicillin

- Class: Antibiotic, Penicillin
- Mechanism of Action: Inhibits bacterial cell wall formation
- Common Uses: Ear infection, sinusitis, strep throat, skin infections
- Memorable Side Effects: GI side effects most common, allergy, rash
- Clinical Pearls:
  - Many patients have an allergy to penicillin; should not be used in patients with a severe allergy (if it is an intolerance like stomach upset, it may be prudent to try a "penicillin" type antibiotic again depending upon the patient's situation)
  - Diarrhea and GI upset are going to be the major/common side effects with penicillin; with mild GI upset and/or diarrhea, hopefully the patient can tough it out and continue therapy
  - Giving penicillin with food or a snack may help reduce GI upset
  - We are going to want to monitor the response of the patient, hopefully they will begin improving by day 2 or 3 of treatment
  - Temperature would be an important thing to monitor for patients who were significantly febrile
  - Usually dosed multiple times throughout the day

Phenazopyridine (Pyridium)

- Class: Urinary Analgesic
- Mechanism of Action: Local anesthetic action in the bladder/urinary tract
- Common Uses: Painful urination (dysuria)
- Memorable Side Effects: GI, dizziness (minimal)
- Clinical Pearls:
  - Very important to identify patients who are taking this and have them assess for infection or something else going on
  - Often will see it used short term for painful urination associated with UTI
  - Not intended for long term use
  - Ensure adequate fluid intake if patient is having UTI's and/or using this medication frequently
  - Can accumulate in kidney disease

Phenytoin (Dilantin)

- Class: Antiepileptic
- Mechanism of Action: Has effects on sodium movement across cells – stabilizes the cell membrane
- Common Uses: Seizures
- Memorable Side Effects: GI, CNS changes, ataxia, vitamin D deficiency, liver function changes (rare)
- Clinical Pearls:
  - Be on the lookout for drug interactions (a few examples: fluconazole, amiodarone, alcohol, cimetidine, fluvoxamine, etc.) – if new meds are started, I would recommend looking up potential interactions
  - Very sensitive to changes in dose (small increase may lead to toxicity)
  - Usual phenytoin level is from 10-20 (can be misleading if patient has low albumin)
  - Toxicity similar to alcohol toxicity in many ways...ataxia (difficulty walking), confusion, GI side effects like nausea, slurred speech, etc.

Pioglitazone (Actos)

- Class: Antidiabetic, TZD
- Mechanism of Action: Improves tissue sensitivity to insulin leading to a reduction in blood glucose
- Common Uses: Diabetes (type 2)
- Memorable Side Effects: Edema, CHF exacerbation, possible elevations in LFT's (rare)
- Clinical Pearls:
  - Usually dosed once daily which is nice
  - If you see a patient on furosemide or other medications that might indicate CHF, pioglitazone is not a good choice as it can worsen edema and exacerbate CHF
  - Monitor for low blood sugar risk, especially in patients on sulfonylureas (i.e. glipizide) or insulins
  - A1C will be important to monitor in any patient on diabetes medications
  - Goal is to keep A1C low and minimize risk of hypoglycemia (this will help decrease risk of diabetes complications like neuropathy, retinopathy, worsening kidney function etc.)

Piperacillin/tazobactam (Zosyn)

- Class: Antibiotic, Penicillin
- Mechanism of Action: Inhibits bacterial cell wall formation
- Common Uses: Broad bacterial coverage (Pseudomonas), Nosocomial pneumonia, reserved for moderate to severe infection
- Memorable Side Effects: GI side effects most common, allergy, rash
- Clinical Pearls:
  - Commonly used for complex bacterial infections
  - Has coverage against Pseudomonas (a common drug resistant hospital infection)
  - Similar to penicillin in chemical structure so have to look out for penicillin, amoxicillin, etc. allergy

Potassium (Klor-Con)

- Class: Potassium Supplement
- Mechanism of Action: Replaces body's potassium
- Common Uses: Low potassium, diuretic use
- Memorable Side Effects: GI side effects (oral), hyperkalemia
- Clinical Pearls:
  - High risk electrolyte as hyperkalemia can cause cardiac arrhythmias
  - Often supplementation is necessary in patients who are on diuretics like furosemide (except potassium sparing diuretics which can increase potassium levels)
  - GI upset is most common and best to take with food
  - With the wax-matrix formulation of potassium, patients may find the outer coating remaining in their stool; the drug is designed to leak out of the matrix shell, educate them that they are getting their potassium (i.e. this is normal and not an issue)
  - Normal potassium level: 3.5-5.1 mEq/L (may vary slightly depending upon lab)
  - By adding ACE Inhibitors, ARBs, or potassium sparing diuretics to the patients medication regimen, we may be able to get away with less potassium supplement
  - Sodium polystyrene sulfonate is used to treat hyperkalemia

Pramipexole (Mirapex)

- Class: Anti-Parkinson's agent, Dopamine Agonist
- Mechanism of Action: Stimulates dopamine receptors
- Common Uses: Restless Legs Syndrome, Parkinson's disorder
- Memorable Side Effects: Orthostasis, edema, OCD symptoms (very rare)
- Clinical Pearls:
  - Indicated for Parkinson's but more commonly drug of choice for RLS
  - Often patients struggle with RLS at night, so if you see it dosed once daily at night, this is likely the indication
  - Keep an eye out for orthostasis, especially in the elderly and patients who may also be receiving numerous antihypertensives already
  - Make sure the medication actually helps the patient, have often seen this added when diagnosis is unclear; cramps versus spasms, versus RLS

Pravastatin (Pravachol)

- Class: Antilipemic, Statin
- Mechanism of Action: HMG Co-A reductase inhibitor (eventually decreases LDL)
- Common Uses: Reduction of cholesterol (particularly LDL)
- Memorable Side Effects: muscle aches, rhabdomyolysis (rare but serious)
- Clinical Pearls:
  - Statins like pravastatin are one of the mainstays of therapy to reduce cholesterol, and more particularly LDL (bad cholesterol)
  - The most notable side effect with statins that you will likely hear patients complain about is myopathy (muscle aches/pain)
  - Usually muscle aches are all over which can help you differentiate from other pain conditions or pain/soreness from an injury or overuse
  - Contraindicated in pregnancy
  - Patients who do not tolerate pravastatin, may try another statin as long as adverse effects aren't too severe (i.e. rhabdomyolysis); if you notice that the patient had an allergy or intolerance, you need to clarify with the provider
  - CPK will be the primary lab to test for rhabdomyolysis – breakdown of muscle; this elevation in CPK may eventually lead to kidney failure
  - Pravastatin tends to have less drug interactions than other statins (atorvastatin, simvastatin, etc.) with CYP3A4 inhibitors like fluconazole or erythromycin

- For most (not all) statins it is "recommended" to give them at night – this is not an absolute, but the drugs ideally work the best when given at night
- Pravastatin is used less frequently because it doesn't reduce LDL as much as newer statins like atorvastatin, simvastatin, and rosuvastatin

Prednisone (Deltasone)

- Class: Corticosteroid
- Mechanism of Action: Suppresses leukocytes and ultimately reduces inflammation, suppresses adrenal function and the immune system
- Common Uses: Many different uses - acute inflammatory states usually most common use (dermatitis, arthritis flare, Crohn's, pneumonia, asthma exacerbation etc.)
- Memorable Side Effects: GI side effects, insomnia, hyperglycemia, long term use; suppress immune system, increase osteoporosis risk as well as cause adrenal insufficiency
- Clinical Pearls:
  - Be sure to take steroids with food as they can be pretty hard on the stomach
  - In patients with diabetes, educate them that a fluctuation in blood sugar may occur when starting, changing doses, or discontinuing this medication due to the adverse effect of hyperglycemia
  - Long term corticosteroid use can lead to increased risk Cushing's (moon face), diabetes, and osteoporosis; make sure long term use is assessed frequently to minimize duration of use and dose of steroids
  - In patients on long term use, they should be assessed if vitamin D and/or calcium and bisphosphonates should be added to reduce osteoporosis risk
  - Insomnia is common in the short term, but may resolve as short term use goes to longer term use
  - Short "bursts" (3 days to a week or 2) are often used to relieve acute inflammatory states causing patient distress (asthma, rheumatoid arthritis, etc.)

- o Corticosteroids (especially long term and higher doses) can also suppress the immune system

Pregabalin (Lyrica)

- Class: Antiepileptic, Analgesic
- Mechanism of Action: Inhibits excitatory neurotransmitters by binding voltage gated calcium channels in the CNS
- Common Uses: Neuropathy, fibromyalgia, seizures
- Memorable Side Effects: Edema, sedation, dizziness, confusion
- Clinical Pearls:
  - Think similar side effect/treatment profile as gabapentin (more expensive, but may be more effective when higher doses are needed)
  - Generally classified as an anti-seizure medication, but often used for neuropathy
  - Keep an eye out for patients with kidney disease who may be experiencing side effects as this drug can accumulate in patients with poor renal function
  - Watch out for dizziness and sedation in our elderly patients as this can potentially contribute to falls
  - Weight gain in the form of edema may potentially happen with gabapentin; be on the lookout for patients with a history CHF and edema issues, as well as those who may already be receiving diuretics like furosemide

Promethazine (Phenergan)

- Class: Antiemetic, Dopamine Blocker, Antihistamine
- Mechanism of Action: Blocks dopamine receptors as well as H1 receptors (antiemetic effects, sedation)
- Common Uses: nausea/vomiting, motion sickness
- Memorable Side Effects: Sedation, fall risk, orthostatic BP changes, EPS, metabolic syndrome
- Clinical Pearls:
  - While promethazine is classically considered an antipsychotic (blocks dopamine), it is most often used for its antiemetic effect
  - Promethazine also has antihistamine effects, which leads to its sedative type effects, and also its ability to be used for allergy type symptoms
  - If promethazine is used on a regular basis, we need to monitor for development of tardive dyskinesia; this is normally not an issue as usually promethazine is used short term and as needed for nausea/vomiting
  - When using injectable forms which can obviously be beneficial for nausea and vomiting to avoid the oral route, the preferred route of administration is intramuscular (into deep muscle)
  - Sedation, orthostatic hypotension, movement disorder side effects can all increase the risk of falls especially in our elderly patients

Propofol (Diprivan)

- Class: Anesthetic
- Mechanism of Action: Possible agonist activity on GABA and blockade of NMDA
- Common Uses: Anesthesia (intubated/ICU type patients)
- Memorable Side Effects: Hypotension, respiratory apnea, elevated triglycerides, respiratory acidosis
- Clinical Pearls:
  - Infusion contains lipids (explains the possibility for elevated triglycerides)
  - Rare risk for anaphylaxis
  - Can be riskier in patients who already have lower blood pressure
  - Very fast onset (less than 1 minute)

Propranolol (Inderal LA)

- Class: Antihypertensive, Beta-blocker
- Mechanism of Action: Blocks beta receptors leading to lower pulse/BP
- Common Uses: Hypertension, atrial fibrillation, migraines, tremor, variceal hemorrhage in patients with cirrhosis (prophylaxis)
- Memorable Side Effects: Low pulse, low BP, fatigue
- Clinical Pearls:
  - Trick to remembering beta receptors: You have 1 heart and 2 lungs (beta-1 is primarily on the heart and beta-2 primarily in the lungs) – non selective beta blockers can contribute to airway restriction (beta-2) as well as lower cardiac output (beta-1)
  - The selectivity of these drugs is really important. Propranolol is the classic example of a beta blocker that is not selective for beta-1 receptors. It also blocks beta-2 receptors which makes it more likely that it could potentially exacerbate respiratory conditions like asthma
  - Propranolol has a unique use of migraine prophylaxis as well as being used for portal hypertension in patients with cirrhosis, tremor, and possibly stress/anxiety type issues
  - Often in practice, providers will place a hold order on beta-blockers if the pulse is too low, and this is done to reduce the risk of significant bradycardia

Pseudoephedrine (Sudafed)

- Class: Decongestant
- Mechanism of Action: Stimulates alpha receptors causing vasoconstriction (beneficial in the respiratory tract)
- Common Uses: Nasal congestion
- Memorable Side Effects: hypertension, urinary retention (watch out for BPH patients), dry mouth, anxiety
- Clinical Pearls:
  - Watch out for elderly/patients at high risk for cardiovascular problems as it can raise BP
  - Can exacerbate BPH
  - Can cause/worsen insomnia and/or anxiety
  - Use is restricted in the U.S. – need to sign a log book to obtain it from the pharmacist; component necessary for making methamphetamine

Quetiapine (Seroquel)

- Class: Antipsychotic
- Mechanism of Action: Blocks dopamine receptors
- Common Uses: Schizophrenia, Bipolar disorder, dementia related behaviors like aggression, hallucinations, delusions (off-label)
- Memorable Side Effects: Sedation, fall risk, orthostatic BP changes, EPS, metabolic syndrome
- Clinical Pearls:
  - Usually higher doses are required for younger patients with schizophrenia and/or bipolar disorder while lower doses can and should be used in the elderly
  - Remember with antipsychotic medications that they block dopamine and can exacerbate conditions where there is a shortage of dopamine like Parkinson's disorder (remember that we use dopamine to treat Parkinson's – i.e. carbidopa/levodopa or pramipexole)
  - Sedation, orthostatic hypotension, movement disorder side effects can all increase the risk of falls especially in our elderly patients
  - NMS (neuroleptic malignant syndrome) is a very rare but very serious complication with antipsychotic medications; a few symptoms of NMS include: fever, hyperreflexia, confusion, delirium, tremor
  - Antipsychotics increase risk of metabolic syndrome (diabetes, elevated lipids, weight gain etc.) – it is important to periodically monitor for this, especially in younger patients with schizophrenia and/or bipolar who may be likely to require long term use of higher doses

- Anticholinergic effects are possible as well with antipsychotics, dry eyes, dry mouth, exacerbation of urinary retention (i.e. BPH), constipation (SLUD – can't salivate, lacrimate, urinate or defecate)
- Antipsychotics can contribute to QTc prolongation, which can be especially problematic in patients who are already at risk (i.e. on antiarrhythmic medications)

Quinapril (Accupril)

- Class: Antihypertensive, ACE Inhibitor
- Mechanism of Action: Quinapril inhibits the angiotensin converting enzyme which prevents the production of angiotensin 2. Angiotensin 2 is a potent vasoconstrictor; less angiotensin 2 equates to less vasoconstriction, and lower blood pressure
- Common Uses: Hypertension, acute MI, heart failure
- Common Side Effects: Cough, kidney impairment, low blood pressure, and hyperkalemia
- Clinical Pearls:
  - ACE Inhibitors are notoriously known for causing a dry chronic cough
  - Angiotensin Receptor Blockers (ARBs) are the cousins to the ACE Inhibitors, and are the first line substitute to a patient who has had a cough with an ACE Inhibitor
  - ACE inhibitors can exacerbate kidney impairment as well as contribute to acute renal failure especially in patients who are already on other potential renal toxic medications (i.e. diuretics, NSAIDs, etc.) even though in conditions like heart failure, diuretics and ACE Inhibitors are often used together
  - ACE Inhibitors are a classic cause of elevated potassium levels; if your patient has hyperkalemia, you must make sure the ACE inhibitor has been addressed
  - In some cases, African Americans may not respond to ACE Inhibitors as well as other ethnicities
  - A common mistake I've seen clinicians make is using an ACE Inhibitor with and ARB; this is generally not recommended

- ACE Inhibitors (and ARBs) are frequently used in patients with hypertension and a history of diabetes, stroke, CAD, CKD, and CHF
- Angioedema (swelling of the lips/airway) is classically caused by ACE inhibitors...it is extremely rare, but very serious requiring immediate discontinuation

Rabeprazole (Aciphex)

- Class: PPI
- Mechanism of Action: Inhibits proton pumps in the stomach leading to a less acidic environment
- Common Uses: GERD, ulcer, Barrett's esophagus
- Memorable Side Effects: Usually pretty well tolerated; Long term use: Possibility to increase fracture risk, decrease B12 levels, C. diff risk, low magnesium
- Clinical Pearls:
  - PPI's are the most potent acid blocker on the market
  - PPI's are generally dosed 30 minutes or so before meals – this is a recommendation, not an absolute (example if a patient likes to get up and eat right away upon rising, the medication will still likely be beneficial, but may not have a maximal effect)
  - For some patients PPI's may not work very quickly, i.e. it might take a few days for maximal effect
  - For the above reason, as needed (PRN) PPI's can possibly be effective, but are generally not recommended
  - Use short term if possible due to increased risk of osteoporosis, low magnesium, and B12 deficiency if used long term
  - Most common primary outcome of PPI would be to improve symptoms likely heartburn and stomach from GERD, stomach ulcer, or other related condition
  - Barrett's esophagus, high risk GI medications (i.e. NSAIDs, prednisone), or chronic GI bleed may require indefinite therapy
  - If GI bleed is problematic, monitoring hemoglobin and/or hemoccult might be appropriate to assess possible blood loss

Ramipril (Altace)

- Class: Antihypertensive, ACE Inhibitor
- Mechanism of Action: Ramipril inhibits the angiotensin converting enzyme which prevents the production of angiotensin 2. Angiotensin 2 is a potent vasoconstrictor; less angiotensin 2 equates to less vasoconstriction, and lower blood pressure
- Common Uses: Hypertension, acute MI, heart failure
- Common Side Effects: Cough, kidney impairment, low blood pressure, and hyperkalemia
- Clinical Pearls:
  - ACE Inhibitors are notoriously known for causing a dry chronic cough
  - Angiotensin Receptor Blockers (ARBs) are the cousins to the ACE Inhibitors, and are the first line substitute to a patient who has had a cough with an ACE Inhibitor
  - ACE inhibitors can exacerbate kidney impairment as well as contribute to acute renal failure especially in patients who are already on other potential renal toxic medications (i.e. diuretics, NSAIDs, etc.) even though in conditions like heart failure, diuretics and ACE Inhibitors are often used together
  - ACE Inhibitors are a classic cause of elevated potassium levels; if your patient has hyperkalemia, you must make sure the ACE inhibitor has been addressed
  - In some cases, African Americans may not respond to ACE Inhibitors as well as other ethnicities
  - A common mistake I've seen clinicians make is using an ACE Inhibitor with and ARB; this is generally not recommended

- ACE Inhibitors (or ARBs) are frequently used in patients with hypertension and a history of diabetes, stroke, CAD, CKD, and CHF
- Angioedema (swelling of the lips/airway) is classically caused by ACE inhibitors...it is extremely rare, but very serious requiring immediate discontinuation

Ranitidine (Zantac)

- Class: Histamine-2 blocker
- Mechanism of Action: Blocks histamine 2 receptors (H2 blocker) which results in reduced gastric acid secretion and a higher pH in the stomach
- Common Uses: GERD, heartburn, GI bleed
- Memorable Side Effects: Pretty well tolerated overall (watch out for CNS changes in elderly)
- Clinical Pearls:
  - H2 blockers are cleared by the kidney, so they can accumulate/require dose adjustments in CKD
  - Generally less effective at suppressing stomach acid than PPI's
  - Many available over the counter, inexpensive
  - CNS effects likely more common in elderly, on higher doses, and in patients with kidney disease
  - Generally used before PPI's if something more than Tums (calcium carbonate) is needed in pregnancy

Rifampin (Rifadin)

- Class: Antibiotic
- Mechanism of Action: Inhibits bacterial RNA synthesis
- Common Uses: TB, augmentation in MRSA/osteomyelitis
- Memorable Side Effects: LFT's increased, GI, rash
- Clinical Pearls:
  - Enzyme inducer – notorious for drug interactions like warfarin (causes lower INR when initiated)
  - MRSA activity

Risedronate (Actonel)

- Class: Bisphosphonate
- Mechanism of Action: Inhibits osteoclasts (osteoclasts break down bone)
- Common Uses: Osteoporosis
- Memorable Side Effects: Esophageal ulceration (administration procedure important to decrease this risk), GI side effects in general
- Clinical Pearls:
  - Timing of administration is critical! Take on an empty stomach, usually right away in the morning with 6-8 ounces of plain water 30 minutes prior to any food or drink (that isn't plain water)
  - Have patient remain sitting or standing upright for 30 minutes (this is to reduce the risk of esophageal irritation/ulceration)
  - Absorption will be limited and drug will not be effective if taken with food or other medications
  - After 3-5 years of bisphosphonate use, some lower risk patients may be able to have the medication reassessed for ongoing need and possibly discontinued
  - Osteonecrosis (destruction or dying) of bone of the jaw is extremely rare (patient may be at increased risk if recently had an invasive dental procedure)
  - Be cautious with oral bisphosphonates in patients who already have esophageal or GI related concerns (GI bleed or ulcer history)
  - Always important to assure adequate vitamin D and calcium intake

Risperidone (Risperdal)

- Class: Antipsychotic
- Mechanism of Action: Blocks dopamine receptors
- Common Uses: Schizophrenia, Bipolar disorder, dementia related behaviors like aggression, hallucinations, delusions (off-label)
- Memorable Side Effects: Sedation, fall risk, orthostatic BP changes, EPS, metabolic syndrome
- Clinical Pearls:
  - Usually higher doses are required for younger patients with schizophrenia and/or bipolar disorder while lower doses can and should be used in the elderly
  - Remember with antipsychotic medications that they block dopamine and can exacerbate conditions where there is a shortage of dopamine like Parkinson's disorder (remember that we use dopamine to treat Parkinson's – i.e. carbidopa/levodopa or pramipexole)
  - Sedation, orthostatic hypotension, movement disorder side effects can all increase the risk of falls especially in our elderly patients
  - NMS (neuroleptic malignant syndrome) is a very rare but very serious complication with antipsychotic medications; a few symptoms of NMS include: fever, hyperreflexia, confusion, delirium, tremor
  - Antipsychotics increase risk of metabolic syndrome (diabetes, elevated lipids, weight gain etc.) – it is important to periodically monitor for this, especially in younger patients with schizophrenia and/or bipolar who may be likely to require long term use of higher doses

- Anticholinergic effects are possible as well with antipsychotics - dry eyes, dry mouth, exacerbation of urinary retention (i.e. BPH), constipation (SLUD – can't salivate, lacrimate, urinate or defecate)
- Antipsychotics can contribute to QTC prolongation, which can be especially problematic in patients who are already at risk (i.e. on antiarrhythmic medications)

Rivaroxaban (Xarelto)

- Class: Anticoagulant
- Mechanism of Action: Inhibits clotting factor 10A
- Common Uses: Prevention of stroke in patients with Atrial Fibrillation, DVT/PE prophylaxis or treatment
- Memorable Side Effects: Bleeding
- Clinical Pearls:
  - Is gaining popularity against warfarin
  - Less risk of drug interaction as well as patients do NOT need to do routine INR's
  - With bleed risk being the major side effect, hemoglobin (CBC) is important to monitor
  - Major use of this medication is to prevent or treat blood clots (DVT, PE, Stroke)
  - Expensive $$ is the major downside of rivaroxaban versus warfarin

Ropinirole (Requip)

- Class: Anti-Parkinson's, Dopamine Agonist
- Mechanism of Action: Stimulates dopamine receptors
- Common Uses: RLS, Parkinson's disorder
- Memorable Side Effects: Orthostasis, edema, OCD symptoms (very rare)
- Clinical Pearls:
  - Indicated for Parkinson's but very commonly drug of choice for RLS
  - Often patients struggle with RLS at night, so if you see it dosed once daily at night, this is likely the indication
  - Keep an eye out for orthostasis, especially in the elderly and patients who may also be receiving numerous antihypertensives already
  - Make sure the medication actually helps the patient, have often seen this added when diagnosis is unclear; cramps versus spasms, versus RLS

Rosuvastatin (Crestor)

- Class: Antilipemic, Statin
- Mechanism of Action: HMG Co-A reductase inhibitor (eventually decreases LDL)
- Common Uses: Reduction of cholesterol (particularly LDL)
- Memorable Side Effects: muscle aches, rhabdomyolysis (rare but serious)
- Clinical Pearls:
  - Statins like rosuvastatin are one of the mainstays of therapy to reduce cholesterol, and more particularly LDL (bad cholesterol)
  - The most notable side effect with statins that you will likely hear patients complain about is myopathy (muscle aches/pain)
  - Usually muscle aches are all over which can help you differentiate from other pain conditions or pain/soreness from an injury or overuse
  - Contraindicated in pregnancy
  - Patients who do not tolerate a rosuvastatin, may try another statin as long as adverse effects aren't too severe (i.e. rhabdomyolysis); if you notice that the patient had an allergy or intolerance, you need to clarify with the provider
  - CPK will be the primary lab to test for rhabdomyolysis – breakdown of muscle
  - For most statins it is "recommended" to give them at night – this is not an absolute, but the drugs ideally work the best when given at night; rosuvastatin is an exception to this rule

Sennosides (Senokot)

- Class: Stimulant laxative
- Mechanism of Action: Stimulates GI movement by irritating GI smooth muscle
- Common Uses: Constipation
- Memorable Side Effects: Abdominal pain
- Clinical Pearls:
  - Used to promote bowel movement
  - Often used in treatment/prevention of opioid induced constipation
  - Can be used as needed

Sertraline (Zoloft)

- Class: Antidepressant, SSRI
- Mechanism of Action: SSRI – selective serotonin reuptake inhibitor; increases serotonin in the brain
- Common Uses: Depression, anxiety, PTSD
- Memorable Side Effects: GI side effects (N/V/D), can really cause sedation or activation depending upon the patient, changes in mental status, hyponatremia (rare)
- Clinical Pearls:
  - SSRI's are generally considered the first line medication to treat depression, they are generally well tolerated, and less risky than other antidepressants in the situation of attempted suicide through overdosing on pills
  - Stomach/GI complaints like stomach upset and/or diarrhea are probably the most common adverse effects (sertraline is highest risk for causing diarrhea of all the SSRI's)
  - There may be an increased risk of suicidal thinking when first starting these medications (there is a BOXED warning for this risk)
  - Although not terribly common, hyponatremia (low sodium) is a possible unique side effect with SSRI's and much more likely in patients already prone to hyponatremia – classic example would be patients who are taking diuretics, which can also lower sodium
  - Remember that these drugs are not an immediate fix! In most cases, SSRI's take weeks sometimes months before a patient will start improving; however side effects will be apparent from the start of the medication, making it difficult to coach our patients to continue the medication in the first few weeks after starting it

- SSRI's are used in pregnancy, but the risk versus the benefits need to be assessed on a case by case basis
- SSRI's can decrease libido

Sildenafil (Viagra)

- Class: PDE-5 inhibitor
- Mechanism of Action: Phosphodiesterase Type 5 inhibitor – releases nitric oxide which is necessary for erection
- Common Uses: Erectile dysfunction, pulmonary arterial hypertension
- Memorable Side Effects: Low blood pressure, vision color changes (seeing blue tinges in vision), flushing
- Clinical Pearls:
  - Originally developed as a blood pressure medication; caution patients about risk of low blood pressure
  - Drug interaction with systemic nitrate/nitroglycerine products (advise patients about potential interaction and elevated risk of low blood pressure)
  - Be sure to assess if other medications may be contributing to sexual dysfunction (antidepressants like SSRI's are a classic example)

Simvastatin (Zocor)

- Class: Antilipemic, Statin
- Mechanism of Action: HMG Co-A reductase inhibitor (eventually decreases LDL)
- Common Uses: Reduction of cholesterol (particularly LDL)
- Memorable Side Effects: muscle aches, rhabdomyolysis (rare but serious)
- Clinical Pearls:
  - Statins like simvastatin are one of the mainstays of therapy to reduce cholesterol, and more particularly LDL (bad cholesterol)
  - The most notable side effect with statins that you will likely hear patients complain about is myopathy (muscle aches/pain)
  - Usually muscle aches are all over which can help you differentiate from other pain conditions or pain/soreness from an injury or overuse
  - Contraindicated in pregnancy
  - Patients who do not tolerate a simvastatin, may try another statin as long as adverse effects aren't too severe (i.e. rhabdomyolysis); if you notice that the patient had an allergy or intolerance, you need to clarify with the provider
  - CPK will be the primary lab to test for rhabdomyolysis – breakdown of muscle; this elevation in CPK may eventually lead to kidney failure
  - If they are going to, patients usually will present with myopathy when the medication is first started or increased, but be on the lookout for new medications that can interact with (some) statins like CYP3A4 inhibitor drug interactions with medications like fluconazole or erythromycin (this

will cause drug concentrations in the body to go up potentially leading to toxicity)
- o Amiodarone, amlodipine, diltiazem are a few other common drug interactions with simvastatin that doses should be reduced or monitored for risk of toxicity
- o Gemfibrozil is a cholesterol medication that also interacts with simvastatin – this drug interaction should be addressed with the primary provider
- o For most statins it is "recommended" to give them at night – this is not an absolute, but the drugs ideally work the best when given at night

Sitagliptin (Januvia)

- Class: Antidiabetic, DDP-4 inhibitor
- Mechanism of Action: Inhibits DPP-4 which increases incretin levels (incretin increases insulin and decreases glucagon in the body and also might help patients' stomachs "feel full")
- Common Uses: Diabetes (type 2)
- Memorable Side Effects: GI (usually pretty well tolerated); pancreatitis and cardiovascular concerns exist, but are rare
- Clinical Pearls:
  - Usually fairly well tolerated, once daily dosing is nice for a diabetes medication
  - Watch out for dose adjustment and accumulation in CKD
  - Usually second or third choice following metformin and/or sulfonylurea in the management of type 2 diabetes (dependent upon how much A1C lowering is necessary)
  - Can be found in combination with metformin (1 pill) – Janumet

Spironolactone (Aldactone)

- Class: Antihypertensive, Potassium Sparing Diuretic, Aldosterone antagonist
- Mechanism of Action: Aldosterone antagonist – increases water excretion and sodium (diuretic) but spares potassium (can increase potassium levels)
- Common Uses: Heart failure, cirrhosis with ascites
- Memorable Side Effects: hyperkalemia, gynecomastia, low BP, hyponatremia, dehydration
- Clinical Pearls:
  - Much like all diuretics, in relation to the effects on the kidney, the risk of overdiuresis (promoting too much fluid loss) is worsening kidney function by inadequate flow through the kidney
  - The development of "moobs" (man boobs) and breast tenderness can be very troubling for male patients on spironolactone (gynecomastia)
  - We can often reduce the potassium supplementation (especially patients on high doses of KCl supplements) burden by using potassium sparing diuretics

Sumatriptan (Imitrex)

- Class: Anti-migraine, Triptan
- Mechanism of Action: Serotonin 5HT agonist – which causes vasoconstriction and reduction in inflammation associated with migraine
- Common Uses: Acute relief of migraine
- Memorable Side Effects: Dizziness, changes in CNS
- Clinical Pearls:
  - Meant for acute relief of migraine, not prophylaxis
  - Comes in multiple formulations (not just oral), injection, nasal, etc. as some may struggle with nausea when they have a migraine
  - Be sure to assess frequent use, if using frequently, need to have control of migraines assessed and have controller medication added (valproic acid, propranolol, topiramate, etc.)
  - Often used with NSAIDs (i.e. naproxen) in migraine treatment
  - Does have serotonin activity so could potentially contribute to serotonin syndrome (higher risk in patients already on SSRI's, tramadol etc.)

Tamsulosin (Flomax)

- Class: Alpha Blocker
- Mechanism of Action: Blocks alpha receptors causing smooth muscle relaxation and opening of the ureter
- Common Uses: BPH, urinary obstruction
- Memorable Side Effects: Low BP, dizziness
- Clinical Pearls:
    - Usually dosed at night to try to avoid/minimize orthostasis risk
    - More selective for the prostate than other alpha blockers, (i.e. terazosin or doxazosin) so less risk of lowering blood pressure
    - Anticholinergics and pseudoephedrine can worsen BPH causing the initiation or increase of alpha blockers like tamsulosin
    - May also be used to help patients pass a ureteral stone, relaxes the smooth muscle and opens up the ureter to ease flow

Temazepam (Restoril)

- Class: Benzodiazepine
- Mechanism of Action: enhances activity of GABA (an inhibitor neurotransmitter that causes sedation)
- Common Uses: Insomnia
- Memorable Side Effects: sedation, confusion, fall risk, dizziness,
- Clinical Pearls:
  - Typically ONLY used for insomnia (not anxiety or seizures)
  - The best way I remember benzodiazepines is that they are very close to "alcohol in a pill"
  - Sedation, confusion, slurred speech, trouble walking (ataxia), etc. are all common with benzo's/alcohol
  - Be cautious with patients on higher doses of benzodiazepines to make sure they aren't abruptly stopped
  - Educate patients on driving/operating machinery risks
  - Falls in the elderly are a big downside to using these medications
  - Benzo's are a controlled substance, i.e. they can cause addiction, etc.
  - Flumazenil is antidote in overdose

Terazosin (Hytrin)

- Class: Antihypertensive, Alpha Blocker
- Mechanism of Action: Blocks alpha receptors causing smooth muscle relaxation, vasodilation, and opening of the ureter
- Common Uses: BPH, urinary obstruction, hypertension
- Memorable Side Effects: Low BP, dizziness
- Clinical Pearls:
    - Non-selective alpha blocker, so can be used for both hypertension and BPH
    - Risk of orthostasis higher with a non-selective alpha blockers like terazosin
    - In the case of worsening urinary retention due to BPH and initiation of these agents, be sure to assess if your patient is on anticholinergic medications (diphenhydramine, TCA's, etc.)
    - Usually dosed at night to minimize the risk of orthostasis

Testosterone (Androgel, Androderm)

- Class: Androgen
- Mechanism of Action: Testosterone hormone - responsible for development of male sex organs, and causes muscle growth
- Common Uses: Testosterone deficiency, metastatic breast cancer
- Memorable Side Effects: Gynecomastia, hypertension, acne, mood changes
- Clinical Pearls:
  - Drug of abuse in sports (increases muscle mass, etc.)
  - Controlled substance – schedule 3 for above reason
  - Testosterone can "amp" you up...think of "Roid Rage" – increased BP, irritability, mood swings, anger, etc.
  - Risk of DVT a possibility (rare)
  - Increase in PSA and possible impotence especially with prolonged use

Tiotropium (Spiriva)

- Class: Inhaled Anticholinergic
- Mechanism of Action: Inhaled anticholinergic can open up airways and decrease secretions
- Common Uses: COPD
- Memorable Side Effects: Dry mouth, cough, irritation to the lungs (usually pretty well tolerated) usually not clinically significant systemic absorption
- Clinical Pearls:
  - Tiotropium is primarily used for COPD, and because it has anticholinergic activity, it can help dry up the airways as well as open them up to allow for better breathing in patients who have think mucous/sputum
  - It is long acting and meant to be used as a controller medication
  - It will not provide acute relief from respiratory distress, not meant to be a rescue inhalation product
  - Often by using this medication in COPD, our goal is likely to improve respiratory status, but also to reduce the amount of as needed albuterol and/or albuterol/ipratropium (Duoneb or Combivent)
  - Tiotropium comes with a special delivery device and capsules; to prepare the device for use, the capsules are inserted into the device and punctured for the contents to be inhaled by the patient
  - With the delivery device, it is imperative to assess if patients are able to adequately coordinate how to use the device as well as if they are able to inhale quickly and forcefully enough to get the drug into their lungs

- Systemic anticholinergic effects (can't spit, see, pee or poop) are usually not a concern as systemic absorption is low

Tolterodine (Detrol LA)

- Class: Bladder Anticholinergic
- Mechanism of Action: Blocks muscarinic receptors (anticholinergic medication) in the bladder which increases urine volume in the bladder and potentially decreases frequency/urge
- Common Uses: Overactive bladder, bladder spasms
- Memorable Side Effects: Anticholinergic effects possible (i.e. dry mouth, dry eyes, urinary retention, constipation)
- Clinical Pearls:
  o Anticholinergic effects
  o Tolterodine is less likely to cause anticholinergic effects than older bladder agents like oxybutynin as it is more selective for the bladder
  o Long acting product available, nice for once daily dosing
  o Be sure to assess if the medication is working for incontinence/frequency
  o Keep an eye out for patients on diuretics and if frequency is the major issue, make sure that diuretics are at the minimum effective dose (not always possible to reduce diuretics with CHF history etc.)
  o Frequency can be especially problematic in patients who have an active social life as well as night when trying to sleep

Topiramate (Topamax)

- Class: Antiepileptic
- Mechanism of Action: Not well understood; possible effects on sodium channels as well as GABA receptors
- Common Uses: Seizures, migraines
- Memorable Side Effects: "Dopamax, Topamax" – can cause cognitive impairment, sedation
- Clinical Pearls:
  - Cognitive slowing is probably the most concerning adverse effect for patients
  - With the indication of migraines being a common issue with women of child-bearing age, be sure to remember that topiramate can reduce the effects of estrogen containing birth control
  - Used for migraine prophylaxis, NOT acute relief
  - With any medication being used to treat seizures, it is very important to not abruptly stop a medication unless there is a very good reason (serious side effect etc.)
  - Weight loss could potentially be a beneficial adverse effect in an overweight seizure or migraine patient

Tramadol (Ultram)

- Class: Opioid, Analgesic
- Mechanism of Action: Binds opioid receptors inhibiting CNS pain pathways and causes pain relief
- Common Uses: Management of pain disorders, both chronic and acute
- Memorable Side Effects: Constipation, sedation, respiratory depression, CNS effects like confusion, delirium etc., increase seizure risk
- Clinical Pearls:
  - Has opioid like effects, so this medication is going to be a potential risk for abuse, drug diversion, addiction, etc.
  - Tramadol is notoriously known for lowering seizure threshold (increasing risk of seizure); if you see a patient who has a seizure diagnosis or is on seizure medications, be sure that the risk versus benefit of tramadol is addressed
  - Confusion, GI upset, constipation, lethargy can be problematic especially in our elderly population (there is a lower recommended maximum dose in the elderly – 300 mg versus 400 mg daily)
  - Naloxone is reversal agent for opioids
  - Can be used on an as needed basis as this medication works fairly quickly
  - It is not as highly controlled by the DEA as other medications in the opioid class (i.e. fentanyl, oxycodone, morphine) – It is a schedule 4 controlled substance where fentanyl etc. are schedule 2 controlled substances
  - Can be given in combination with non-opioid analgesics like acetaminophen
  - Tramadol can increase the risk of serotonin syndrome, and this is especially true at higher doses

and patients who are already receiving other medications that can increase serotonin (i.e. SSRI's or SNRI's)

Travoprost (Travatan)

- Class: Prostaglandin
- Mechanism of Action: Prostaglandin F2 alpha analog – decreases intraocular pressure
- Common Uses: Glaucoma
- Memorable Side Effects: Change in eye color, eye irritation
- Clinical Pearls:
  - Change in eye color may be permanent (change to brown)
  - Many glaucoma patients will be on multiple eye drops – at least 5 minutes is the appropriate amount of time to wait between drops

Trazodone (Desyrel)

- Class: Antidepressant
- Mechanism of Action: Inhibits reuptake of serotonin, but differs from SSRI's in that it has blocking activity on H1 and alpha 1 receptors (H1 blocking activity gives this medication its sedative properties)
- Common Uses: Sleep, depression
- Memorable Side Effects: Sedation, dizziness, orthostasis
- Clinical Pearls:
  - While it is usually classified as an antidepressant, trazodone at lower doses is most frequently used for insomnia
  - Usually the antidepressant benefits of trazodone are seen at higher doses
  - Must educate patients on its sedative properties and risk of driving, etc.
  - Trazodone can be used "prn" or as needed for sleep, but you should never see it used as needed for depression as it usually takes significant time (like SSRI's) for the antidepressant effect to begin
  - Keep an eye out for postural hypotension (dizziness upon rising) especially in our elderly patients and those already on blood pressure lowering medications – if you remember from the mechanism of action above, it does have alpha blocking activity
  - Trazodone can contribute to dry mouth, be on the lookout for patients who complain about this or are using saliva substitute medications (example: Biotene)

Triamcinolone (Kenalog)

- Class: Topical Corticosteroid
- Mechanism of Action: Suppresses mediators of inflammation (histamine, kinins, prostaglandins etc.) resulting in less inflammation/redness
- Common Uses: Dermatitis
- Memorable Side Effects: local irritation - systemic side effects can happen; prolonged use, large areas obviously increase risk of adrenal suppression, HPA-axis suppression, etc.
- Clinical Pearls:
  o If patients don't see improvement in condition in 1-2 weeks, be sure they know to get reassessed
  o Long term use (especially if large amounts/areas of the body can lead to significant systemic absorption) can suppress the HPA axis
  o Long term use probably more concerning in young children
  o Systemic problems not likely if used short term

Triamterene/HCTZ (Dyazide)

- Class: Triamterene – Potassium Sparing Diuretic; HCTZ – See Hydrochlorothiazide
- Mechanism of Action: Triamterene is a potassium sparing diuretic that blocks sodium channels in the kidney; hydrochlorothiazide is a thiazide diuretic
- Common Uses: Hypertension, edema
- Memorable Side Effects: Triamterene (hyperkalemia), HCTZ (hypokalemia), dehydration (rising creatinine and BUN), low blood pressure, orthostasis risk, electrolyte imbalances
- Clinical Pearls:
    - Much like all diuretics, in relation to the effects on the kidney, the risk of overdiuresis is worsening kidney function
    - We can often reduce the potassium supplementation (especially patients on high doses of KCl supplements) burden by using potassium sparing diuretics
    - Triamterene, while generally lumped into the group of potassium sparing diuretics because it causes elevations in potassium, does have a slightly different mechanism of action – it acts on sodium channels in the late distal convoluted tubule; it doesn't compete with aldosterone like spironolactone
    - Patients often forget they are actually on two medications when they are used in combination in one pill
    - See HCTZ (hydrochlorothiazide) alone for its clinical pearls

Trimethoprim/sulfamethoxazole (Bactrim)

- Class: Antibiotic
- Mechanism of Action: Sulfamethoxazole inhibits bacterial folic acid production which trimethoprim essentially does the same via a different mechanism
- Common Uses: UTI, URI's, PCP (common in HIV patients)
- Memorable Side Effects: GI, rash, CNS changes
- Clinical Pearls:
  - Very common treatment for UTI
  - Sulfa allergy is common in many patients! Look out!
  - Major drug interaction with warfarin (increases INR)
  - Has some activity against MRSA
  - Trimethoprim can increase risk for hyperkalemia in patients on ACEI's, ARB's, Potassium supplements, and Potassium Sparing Diuretics

Valacyclovir (Valtrex)

- Class: Antiviral
- Mechanism of Action: Converted to acyclovir which inhibits DNA synthesis and viral replication
- Common Uses: Shingles, Genital herpes, chicken pox
- Memorable Side Effects: GI most common, CNS side effects more likely in elderly and/or poor kidney function
- Clinical Pearls:
  - Typically for most viral infections (and bacterial for that matter), the sooner treatment is started once an infection is identified, the better
  - You can think of acyclovir and valacyclovir as the same...the big advantage of valacyclovir is that patients don't need to take it so many times per day
  - Monitor for GI side effects, and Liver Function Tests will be more important if long term use is necessary
  - May need to reduce dose and/or have a heightened awareness for potential adverse effects in patients with poor kidney function

Valsartan (Diovan)

- Class: Antihypertensive, ARB
- Mechanism of Action: Blocks the angiotensin 2 receptor – ends up preventing vasoconstriction, aldosterone release etc. (remember aldosterone antagonists can raise potassium just like ARBs and ACE Inhibitors)
- Common Uses: hypertension, heart failure
- Memorable Side Effects: hyperkalemia, exacerbate/worsen kidney function, low blood pressure
- Clinical Pearls:
  - When you think of ARBs and ACE inhibitors, you can lump the side effects together as they are overall the same
  - One major exception to the above rule is the side effect of cough; cough usually doesn't happen with ARBs, and in many patients you will see patients who develop cough on an ACE inhibitor be transitioned to an ARB
  - Kidney function changes and monitoring of potassium is critical when doses are changed or an ARB is initiated
  - This worsening kidney function risk increases in patients who may be taking NSAIDs and/or diuretics
  - As with any medication used to treat hypertension, we need to educate our patients to rise slowly when getting up to minimize risk of orthostatic (sometimes called postural) hypotension

Vancomycin (Vancocin)

- Class: Antibiotic, Glycopeptide
- Mechanism of Action: Inhibits bacterial cell wall synthesis
- Common Uses: MRSA (methicillin resistant Staph. aureus), orally can be used to treat C. diff
- Memorable Side Effects: hypotension, flushing, red man syndrome (pretty rare now), given orally – GI adverse effects
- Clinical Pearls:
  - Red man syndrome possible if infused too quickly
  - If red man syndrome happens, should be able to slow infusion rate to help treat
  - Trough concentration and kidney function may be important to help guide dosing
  - Drug of choice for methicillin resistant Staph. aureus (MRSA)
  - You should never see this medication taken orally (one exception is a GI infection like C. Diff) – it has poor oral absorption into the blood circulation through the GI tract

Varenicline (Chantix)

- Class: Smoking Cessation Agent
- Mechanism of Action: Partial agonist at nicotine receptors (blocks craving/positive response from nicotine)
- Common Uses: Smoking cessation
- Memorable Side Effects: Abnormal dreams, insomnia, GI, mental health concerns
- Clinical Pearls:
  - Abnormal behavioral and psych issues is a significant problem
  - Vivid or unusual dreams is a significant problem for patients
  - Box warning for depression/suicide, etc.
  - Recommended only to use for 11 weeks
  - Intended to make smoking less rewarding/enjoyable

Vasopressin (Vasostrict)

- Class: Vasoconstrictor
- Mechanism of Action: Causes an increase in cyclic AMP which causes multiple effects including vasoconstriction
- Common Uses: Vasodilation related shock
- Memorable Side Effects: Arrhythmia, MI, heart failure
- Clinical Pearls:
  - Vasoconstrictor used to increase BP (used for vasodilatory shock)
  - Can impact sodium levels
  - BP/Pulse important to monitor

Venlafaxine (Effexor)

- Class: Antidepressant, SNRI
- Mechanism of Action: Selective serotonin and norepinephrine reuptake inhibitor (SNRI)
- Common Uses: Depression, pain syndromes (neuropathy especially)
- Memorable Side Effects: GI side effects, can exacerbate hypertension (usually at higher doses), CNS changes
- Clinical Pearls:
  - Has effects on both serotonin and norepinephrine
  - GI and central nervous system side effects (CNS) will likely be the most common
  - Decreased libido can be an issue for patients taking venlafaxine
  - Be careful with the risk of serotonin syndrome especially in patients on other serotonergic medications
  - Antidepressant effect may take a while to work (weeks)

Verapamil (Calan)

- Class: Antihypertensive, Calcium Channel Blocker
- Mechanism of Action: Blocks calcium channels resulting in vasodilation and cardiac relaxation
- Common Uses: Atrial fibrillation, hypertension
- Memorable Side Effects: Low pulse, low BP, constipation, edema
- Clinical Pearls:
  - Very important distinction: Verapamil and Diltiazem (non-dihydropyridine's) are the calcium channel blockers that act on the heart AND blood vessels; you will not see amlodipine and nifedipine used in atrial fibrillation, because their activity is primarily on the vessels. This also means that pulse monitoring will not be necessary with nifedipine and amlodipine
  - The higher you push the dose on these medications, the more likely you will see the side effect of edema. Keep an eye out for new requirement of diuretic Rx's to treat the edema caused by the calcium channel blockers.
  - Simvastatin is a very common medication that interacts with verapamil
  - Comes in multiple different formulations (long acting, short acting, etc.), make sure you have the right one

Vitamin D

- Class: Vitamin D Derivative
- Mechanism of Action: Vitamin D increases calcium/phosphorus absorption in the gut
- Common Uses: Vitamin supplementation in osteoporosis or vitamin D deficiency (Rickets), hypoparathyroidism
- Memorable Side Effects: Well tolerated at replacement doses (can accumulate if high doses used for a long period of time – fat soluble)
- Clinical Pearls:
    o Most commonly used in patients with osteoporosis history
    o Moving target on what is an adequate goal vitamin D level – most common goal at this point is >30 ng/mL
    o May have some benefit in patients who are frequent fallers
    o Remember that patients in northern climates (less sunlight) may be at higher risk for low levels
    o For maintenance, can simply do daily supplements at lower doses (i.e. 1,000 to 2,000 units), but may also do BIG doses once monthly (50,000 units)

Warfarin (Coumadin, Jantoven)

- Class: Anticoagulant
- Mechanism of Action: Inhibition of clotting factors 2, 7, 9, and 10 – some folks remember this by the term "SNOT" seven, nine, '10', two
- Common Uses: Prevention of blood clots such as DVT, prevention of thromboembolic stroke from atrial fibrillation
- Common Side Effects: Bleeding, purple toe syndrome (rare)
- Clinical Pearls:
  - Warfarin has a ton of drug interactions, antibiotics (sulfamethoxazole/trimethoprim, metronidazole, levofloxacin etc.) being a very common cause of drug interactions; be sure physician is aware/reminded that patients are on warfarin when new medications are started or doses of medications might be changed
  - Bleeding, Bruising, INR, CBC are of highest monitoring importance
  - Vitamin K is the antidote to too much warfarin; ideal way to give vitamin K is orally – also remember that many foods contain vitamin K (green leafy vegetables etc.); diet changes can affect INR, consistency is the key!
  - Younger patients may require doses 10+ mg or greater whereas elderly maybe need as little as 1-2 mg per day
  - Usual goal range INR is 2-3; It is always important to have the goal INR range listed/addressed by the practitioner monitoring warfarin; this allows you to ask questions as to why the dose wasn't changed if the INR falls outside this range

- In patients who are at high risk for bleed, i.e. frequent falls, GI bleed history etc., a lower goal INR may be recommended
- Purple toe syndrome rarely happens likely to the patient being started on too high of an initial dose of warfarin
- Normal GI bacteria also produce vitamin K, changes in the gut bacteria due to antibiotics can also impact the INR

Zolpidem (Ambien)

- Class: "Z" Drug, Sedative
- Mechanism of Action: enhances activity of GABA (an inhibitor neurotransmitter that causes sedation)
- Common Uses: Insomnia
- Memorable Side Effects: sedation, confusion, fall risk, dizziness, abnormal sleep behaviors (sleep walking, eating etc.)
- Clinical Pearls:
  - Often classified as a "Z" drug, medications like zolpidem are sedating; when medications are sedating we always have to be mindful of the morning after and make sure patients realize that driving and/or operating machinery can be extremely dangerous
  - It is recommended to try to use these medications only for short term if possible
  - Sleep hygiene, non-drug interventions are the preferred treatment for insomnia
  - Before these types of medications are prescribed, keep an eye out for patients who may be on stimulating type medications or medications that can contribute to insomnia and make sure that these are assessed prior to giving a sleep medication – classic examples: methylphenidate, prednisone, too much levothyroxine, etc.
  - Zolpidem is a controlled substance in the U.S.; there is a risk of addiction/dependence
  - Very similar effects to benzodiazepines (example: lorazepam)
  - Can greatly increase risk of falls especially in our elderly patients

60 Classes in 60 Minutes

5-Alpha Reductase Inhibitors – Finasteride, Dutasteride

- Primary use: BPH
- Slow onset of benefit
- Shrink prostate, allow improved urine flow
- Adverse effect-impotence

5-HT3 Receptor Antagonists – Ondansetron, Granisetron

- Primary use: Nausea and vomiting
- Used in treatment and prevention (chemotherapy)
- CNS side effects
- QTc prolongation risk

ACE Inhibitors – Lisinopril, Enalapril

- Primary use: Hypertension
- Side Effects – Hyperkalemia, cough, low blood pressure
- Monitor kidney function and potassium
- Angioedema (very rare, but serious)

Acetylcholinesterase Inhibitors – Donepezil, Rivastigmine

- Primary use: Dementia
- Delay progression, doesn't reverse dementia
- GI (N/V/D) side effects, weight loss

Alpha Blockers – Terazo**sin**, Tamsulo**sin**

- Primary use: Hypertension (not tamsulosin), BPH
- Orthostatic Hypotension
- Dosed at night to avoid daytime dizziness/syncope

Aminoglycosides – Tobra**mycin**, Genta**micin**

- Primary use: Gram negative bacterial infections
- IV only (for systemic use)
- Ototoxicity, kidney toxic
- Drug levels are drawn to guide dosing (peak/trough)

Anticoagulants – He**parin**, Enoxa**parin**

- Primary use: Prevention and/or treatment of blood clots
- Injectable only
- Risk of bleed and heparin induced thrombocytopenia (risk much lower with enoxaparin)
- Can be used in short term (unlike warfarin which takes some time to get to therapeutic levels)
- Protamine is antidote

Antiplatelet – Aspirin, Clopido**grel**, Prasu**grel**

- Primary use: Heart Attack (MI), Stroke
- Bleeding risk
- Inhibits platelets from "sticking" together
- Aspirin and Clopidogrel (or Prasugrel) work via different mechanisms, so can be used together

Antipsychotics – Risperi**done**, Paliperi**done**, Quetia**pine,** Olanza**pine** (lots of different endings with antipsychotics, be careful!)

- Primary use: Schizophrenia, Bipolar Disorder
- EPS (movement disorders)
- CNS SE's
- Metabolic Syndrome

ARB's – losartan, valsartan

- Primary use: Hypertension
- Hyperkalemia, low blood pressure risk
- Monitor Kidney Function

Azole Antifungals – ketoconazole, fluconazole

- Primary use: Fungal infection (candida)
- Drug interactions common (CYP 3A4 interactions) – look them up!
- CNS changes, GI SE's, liver function test changes (more rare)

Benzodiazepines – Lorazepam, Clonazepam

- Primary use: Anxiety, Sleep
- Effective as needed
- Sedation
- Falls Risk
- Confusion
- Flumazenil is antidote in overdose

Beta Blockers – metoprolol, carvedilol

- Primary use: Hypertension, Atrial Fibrillation
- Low Pulses, BP monitoring
- Fatigue

Beta-2 Agonists – **Albuterol**, Formo**terol**

- Primary use: Asthma, COPD
- Albuterol – short acting; formoterol, salmeterol – long acting
- Open up the airways
- Don't use long acting for acute relief
- Side effects: Tachycardia, Tremor, Anxiety

Biguanide – Metformin

- Primary use: Diabetes
- Low to zero risk of hypoglycemia when used alone
- GI side effects most common (give with food/meal)
- Risk of lactic acidosis (especially with poor kidney function)

Bisphosphonates – Alen**dronate**, Rise**dronate**

- Primary use: Osteoporosis
- Very important administration procedure – at least 30 minutes before other food/meds/drink, full glass of water, remain upright
- Administration procedure intended to avoid esophageal ulceration, blocking absorption (avoid co-administration with food, meds, other drinks)
- Most dosed once weekly

Calcium Channel Blockers – Amlodi**pine**, Nifedi**pine**, Diltiazem, Verapamil

- Primary use: Hypertension, Atrial Fibrillation
- Edema
- Pulses (Diltiazem and Verapamil) and BP monitoring
- Constipation

Cardiac Glycosides – Digoxin

- Primary use – Atrial fibrillation, CHF
- Toxicity – usually levels >2 (GI, low pulse, CNS changes, weight loss, visual changes)
- CHF lower levels needed than A fib
- Use with caution in elderly and kidney disease (drug can accumulate)

Cephalosporins – **Ceph**alexin, **Cef**triaxone

- Primary use: Bacterial infection (URI, skin very common)
- Multiple generations of cephalosporin medications (in general, higher generations cover more bacteria)
- GI side effects
- Somewhat similar structure to penicillin's, low risk of cross reactivity if allergic to one or the other, but possible

COX-2 Inhibitors – Cele**coxib**

- Primary use: Pain, Inflammation
- Less GI Bleeding (but still can cause) than traditional NSAIDs
- Edema, CHF, Kidney function SE's remain
- Boxed Warning – MI and Stroke Risk

Dipeptidyl Peptidase-4 Inhibitors – Sita**gliptin**, Saxa**gliptin**

- Primary use: Diabetes
- Less hypoglycemia and weight gain than sulfonylureas
- Helps increase incretin hormone which promotes fullness
- Pretty well tolerated, GI most prominent

DMARDs – Methotrexate, Sulfasalazine

- Primary use: Inflammatory diseases (i.e. rheumatoid arthritis)
- Suppress immune system, infection risk
- Methotrexate dosed once weekly
- Methotrexate and Sulfasalazine can impact folic acid, liver function

Dopamine Agonists – Ropinir**ole**, Pramipex**ole**

- Primary use: Restless Legs Syndrome, Parkinson's
- Orthostatic hypotension
- CNS SE's
- GI SE's
- Rare – Obsessive/compulsive type behaviors (i.e. gambling)

Erythropoiesis Stimulating Agents – erythro**poietin**, darbe**poetin**

- Primary use: Treatment of Anemia
- Hypertension
- Risk of MI, Stroke
- Iron supplementation may be necessary

Gaba Drugs – Pre**gaba**lin, **Gaba**pentin

- Primary use: Neuropathy, Pain
- Sedation, Dizziness
- Edema
- Can accumulate in poor kidney function

H1 Blockers, First Generation – Diphenhydram**ine**, Hydroxyz**ine (careful with this ending – very common in multiple drug classes, i.e. clozapine, ranitidine, clonidine etc.)**

- Primary use: Sleep, Allergies, Anxiety
- Anticholinergic effects (Can't spit, see, pee, poop)
- Sedation
- Fall and CNS effects (especially elderly)

Histamine Receptor 2 Blockers – Ranitid**ine**, Famotid**ine (be careful with ending again)**

- Primary use: Heartburn, GERD, GI ulcer
- Quicker onset, but generally considered less effective than PPI's
- Dose adjustment with poor kidney function
- CNS effects especially with elderly or kidney disease

HMG-CoA Inhibitors (Statins) – Simva**statin**, Atorva**statin**

- Primary use: High cholesterol (LDL primarily)
- Muscle pain (myopathy)
- Rhabdomyolysis (rare, but serious – CPK is lab to check)
- Many recommended to be dosed at night

Inhaled Anticholinergics – Tio**tropium**, Ipra**tropium**

- Primary use: COPD
- Ipratropium is short acting (can use as needed) vs. tiotropium long acting
- Dry mouth most common, very little systemic absorption

Long acting insulins – Glargine, Detemir

- Primary use: Lower blood sugar
- Often called "basal" – usually dosed once daily to lower blood sugars all day (occasionally may see twice daily at higher doses)
- Hypoglycemia risk with any insulin product
- Watch out for low fasting blood sugar in the morning
- Glucagon is antidote for severe hypoglycemia

Loop Diuretics – Furosem**ide**, Torsem**ide**, Bumetan**ide** (again, careful with the ending, i.e. hydrochlorothiazide, liraglutide)

- Primary use: Edema, CHF
- Electrolyte Imbalances (hypokalemia) – may require supplementation of potassium
- Dehydration – monitor kidney function
- Urinary Frequency
- Low blood pressure

Macrolides – Azithro**mycin**, Erythro**mycin**, Clarithro**mycin** (careful with ending again – tobramycin, vancomycin etc.)

- Primary use: Bacterial infection – URI, bronchitis, ear infection, etc. (usually an alternative to penicillin antibiotics)
- Erythromycin, Clarithromycin seldom used (drug interactions)
- Azithromycin has a longer half-life, less frequent dosing is nice
- GI adverse effects most common

Miscellaneous Analgesic – Acetaminophen

- Usual drug of choice in elderly, pregnancy for generalized pain
- Not many drug interactions
- Pretty well tolerated, liver toxicity is risk with overdose
- Acetylcysteine is antidote

New Oral Anticoagulants (NOACs) – Rivaroxab**an**, Apixab**an**, Dabigatr**an**

- Primary use: Post op clot prevention, Stroke prevention in A Fib, DVT treatment or prophylaxis
- Bleed risk
- No INR necessary (different from warfarin)

Newer Seizure Meds – Levetiracetam, Lamotrigine

- Sedation, CNS changes most common SE's
- Lamotrigine – rash risk
- Some interactions with lamotrigine, but generally less with these two than older seizure meds like phenytoin, carbamazepine
- May see lamotrigine for mood disorders (bipolar)

Nitrates – Isosorbide mono**nitrate**, **Nitro**glycerine

- Primary use: Angina, Hypertension
- Orthostasis risk
- Sublingual most common for acute relief of chest pain
- Nitrate tolerance risk with chronic use

NMDA Antagonist – Memantine **(careful with ending)**

- Primary use: Dementia

- Delay progression, doesn't reverse dementia
- CNS adverse effects

Non-Steroidal Anti Inflammatory Drugs – Ibuprofen, Naproxen (aspirin can be classified here as well)

- Primary use: Pain, Fever, Inflammation (aspirin – cardiovascular prophylaxis)
- GI upset/pain, GI ulcer (take with food)
- Kidney function monitoring
- CHF exacerbation risk

Older Seizure Meds – Phenytoin, Carbamazepine

- Cause a bunch of drug interactions (enzyme inducers which can reduce concentrations of many drugs)
- Liver monitoring important
- Sometimes can cause rash issues
- Phenytoin total level usually 10-20 (free level 1-2), Carbamazepine 4-12
- Toxicity – CNS changes like confusion and sedation, fall risk (ataxia), GI (similarities to alcohol toxicity)

Opioids – Oxycodone, Hydromorphone, Morphine, Fentanyl

- Primary use: Pain
- Constipation
- Drugs of Abuse
- CNS effects, sedation, respiratory depression
- Naloxone is antidote/reversal agent

Penicillin's – Amoxicillin, Ampicillin

- Primary use: Bacterial infection (URI, skin very common)
- Pediatric use common, ear infection, strep throat etc.

- Diarrhea/GI SE's – can give with food
- Be aware of potential class allergy if patient is allergic to one (rash)
- Used in pregnancy

Potassium Sparing Diuretics – Spironolact**one**, Epleren**one**, Triamterene

- Primary use: Edema, CHF, Hypertension
- Hyperkalemia
- Monitor Kidney Function
- Gynecomastia - spironolactone

Prostaglandins – Latanoprost, Bimatoprost, Travoprost

- Primary use: Glaucoma
- Eye color changes possible
- At least 5 minutes (some will say up to 10 especially if different kind of drops) between drops

Proton Pump Inhibitors – Ome**prazole**, Panto**prazole**

- Primary use: Heartburn, GERD, GI ulcer
- Short term use recommended if possible
- C Diff and Osteoporosis risk long term
- Often used for prophylaxis of GI bleeding (in hospital and on blood thinning medications and/or NSAIDs)

Quinolones – Levo**floxacin**, Cipro**floxacin**, Moxi**floxacin**

- Primary use: UTI's (cipro, levo), Pneumonia (levo, moxi)
- Usually reserved for more complicated pneumonia
- GI, CNS most common adverse effects
- Dose adjustments with poor kidney function

- Drug interaction with calcium, iron, and magnesium (decreases absorption when co-administered orally – separate timing)

Rapid Acting Insulins – Lispro, Aspart

- Primary use: Treat high blood sugars acutely
- Hypoglycemia risk (especially shortly after administration)
- Often dosed with meals to prevent blood sugar from getting too high right after eating (post-prandial)
- Not ideal, but may see sliding scale (check blood sugar, if high, give a certain number of units based upon how high)
- Glucagon is antidote for severe hypoglycemia

Second Generation Histamine-1 Antagonists – Loratad**ine**, Cetiriz**ine**, Fexofenad**ine (careful with this ending)**

- Primary use: Allergies
- Sedation (less than older antihistamines)
- Anticholinergic effects possible but less than older antihistamines (i.e. diphenhydramine)

Selective Serotonin & Norepinephrine Reuptake Inhibitors (SNRI) – Venlafax**ine**, Duloxet**ine**

- Primary use: Depression, Anxiety, Neuropathy
- GI SE's
- Slow onset of benefit especially for mood disorders
- CNS SE's, sexual dysfunction
- Possibly changes in hypertension/pulse especially at higher doses

Selective Serotonin Reuptake Inhibitors – Sertraline, Citalopram, Escitalopram, Fluoxetine (careful with common ending)

- Primary use: Depression, Anxiety
- GI SE's
- Slow onset of benefit
- CNS SE's
- Sexual dysfunction (reduced libido)

Skeletal Muscle Relaxants – Baclofen, Cyclobenzaprine

- Primary use: Muscle spasms
- Sedation
- Anticholinergic (watch tolerability in elderly)

Stimulant Laxatives – Sennosides, Bisacodyl

- Primary use: Treatment of Constipation
- Can be used as needed
- Used for opioid induced constipation

Stimulants – Methylphenidate, Amphetamines

- Primary use: ADHD
- Weight Loss
- Hypertension
- Tachycardia

Sulfonylureas – Glipizide, Glyburide (careful with this ending)

- Primary use: Diabetes
- Stimulates insulin release
- Hypoglycemia
- Weight Gain

Systemic Corticosteroids – Prednis**one**, Methylprednisol**one**, Prednisol**one** (carful with this ending)

- Primary use: Acute inflammatory disorders (asthma, RA, etc.)
- Long Term Risks – Osteoporosis, Diabetes, Cushing's
- Infection risk (especially higher dose, long term)
- GI SE's – take with food
- Insomnia

Thiazide Diuretics – hydrochlorothiazide, chlorthalid**one**, metolaz**one** (carful with this ending)

- Primary use: Hypertension, Edema
- Electrolytes (hypokalemia important, may require supplement)
- Frequent urination
- Kidney function monitoring
- Increase uric acid (exacerbate gout)

Thyroid supplementation – Levothyroxine

- Primary use: Replacement in patients with hypothyroidism
- Side effects, same as patients who have hyperthyroidism (tachycardia, anxiety, weight loss, insomnia etc.)
- Absorption can be decreased by administration with other drugs/food (calcium is classic example) – consistency is key
- TSH monitoring is most important (dosing is counterintuitive – high TSH - dose increased, low TSH - dose reduced)

Triptans – **Sumatriptan**

- Primary use: Migraines
- Used as needed, give at onset of headache, not intended for prophylaxis
- CNS SE's

Urinary Anticholinergics – Tolterodine, Solifenacin, Oxybutynin

- Primary use: Urinary incontinence, frequency
- Anticholinergic adverse effects (Can't spit, see, pee, poop)
- CNS effects (elderly more problematic)

Vitamin K antagonist – Warfarin

- Primary use: DVT, Stroke prevention with atrial fibrillation, PE
- Drug interactions common (many antibiotics) – look them up!
- Vitamin K is the antidote to warfarin overdose
- Bleed risk – INR's monitored with usual goal in the 2-3 range

Xanthine Oxidase Inhibitors – Allopurinol, Febuxostat

- Primary use: Gout prophylaxis
- Monitor uric acid (should go down)
- Not for acute flare
- Can accumulate in kidney disease (especially allopurinol)

Z-Drugs – Zolpidem, Eszopiclone (have a "Z" in them for sleep!)

- Primary use: Sleep
- Short term use recommended if possible
- Adverse effects similar to benzodiazepines
- Watch out for morning "hangover" type effects